DATE DUE

SEP 13, 2004	
	PRINTED IN U.S.A.

The Watts
Teen
Health
Dictionary

by Charlotte Isler, R.N.
and Alwyn T. Cohall, M.D.

with illustrations by David Kelley

FRANKLIN WATTS
A Division of Grolier Publishing
New York   London   Toronto   Sydney
Danbury, Connecticut

To Werner, Donald, and Norman, who used to be teenagers, and to Nick, who is.

Charlotte Isler

This book is dedicated to my loving wife Renee, and my three terrific sons Janon, Jonathan, and Brandon; and to my parents who helped guide me through the ups and downs of adolescence.

Alwyn T. Cohall

We wish to express our appreciation to our editor, Lorna Greenberg, whose tireless efforts have helped to make this book a truly reader-friendly resource for adolescents looking for answers to urgent questions about teen health and life.

Charlotte Isler   *Alwyn T. Cohall*

Interior book design and pagination: Carole Desnoes

Library of Congress Cataloging-in-Publication Data

Isler, Charlotte.
    The Watts teen health dictionary / by Charlotte Isler and Alwyn T. Cohall; illustrated by David Kelley.
        p.   cm.
    Includes bibliographical references and index.
    Summary: Uses the dictionary form to present information about health. Includes appendixes on hotlines, medications, street drugs, health care specialists, and other suggested reading materials.
    ISBN 0-531-11236-5 (LIB.BOG.); 0-531-15792-X (PBK.)
    1. Medicine, Popular—Dictionaries, Juvenile.   2. Health—Dictionaries, Juvenile.
3. Teenagers.   [1. Medicine—Dictionaries. 2. Health—Dictionaries. 3. Teenagers.]
I. Cohall, Alwyn T. II. Kelley, David, 1992– ill. III. Title.
RC81.A2I84   1995
610'.835—dc20   95-22166
                                                                       CIP AC

CONTENTS

FOREWORD

Do you ever have questions like these: What is safe sex? Are my breasts the right size? Is my penis too small? What is a sexually transmitted disease (infection)? You'll find the answers to these and many other urgent questions right here, from A to Z.

If you need help or advice in a hurry, Appendix A lists several hotlines. You'll also find a guide to drugs used in teen health care, a section on street drugs, a First Aid guide, and other important and useful information.

Keep your *Teen Health Dictionary* close by. There'll be many times you'll want some answers and reliable facts, and we hope you'll find what you need here.

Charlotte Isler, R.N.   Alwyn T. Cohall, M.D.

The Watts
Teen
Health
Dictionary

The Human Body FEMALE

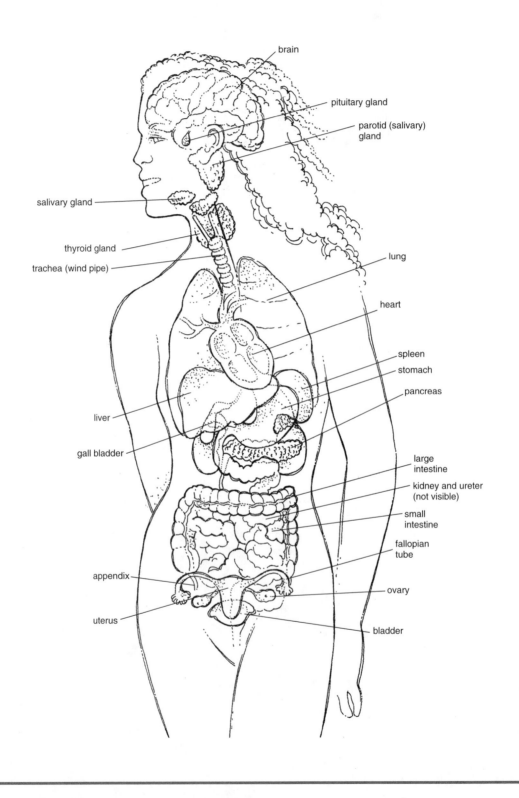

brain

pituitary gland

parotid (salivary) gland

salivary gland

thyroid gland

trachea (wind pipe)

lung

heart

spleen

stomach

pancreas

liver

gall bladder

large intestine

kidney and ureter (not visible)

small intestine

fallopian tube

appendix

ovary

uterus

bladder

The Human Body MALE

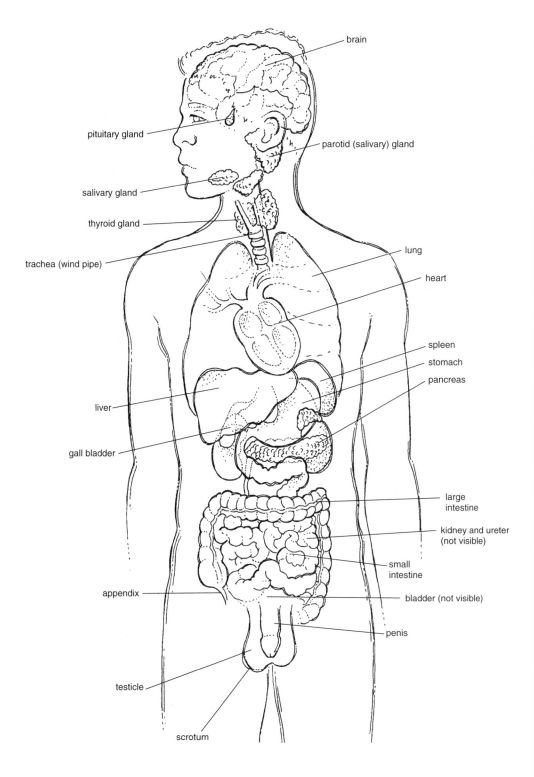

brain

pituitary gland

parotid (salivary) gland

salivary gland

thyroid gland

lung

trachea (wind pipe)

heart

spleen

stomach

pancreas

liver

gall bladder

large intestine

kidney and ureter (not visible)

small intestine

appendix

bladder (not visible)

penis

testicle

scrotum

The Teen Health Dictionary From A to Z

A

Abasia. The inability to walk normally due to poor muscular coordination.

Abdomen (belly). The part of the trunk that extends from below the chest to the bottom of the pelvic area. The abdominal cavity contains many vital organs, including the stomach, liver, spleen, gallbladder, and the intestines.

Abdominal pain. Discomfort or pain in the region between the chest and the pubic area that may be caused by indigestion, diarrhea, or stress. Abdominal pain that continues or gets worse may be a sign of a more serious problem, such as an intestinal disease, or one that requires surgery, such as acute appendicitis. In girls, lower abdominal pain may indicate a problem in the reproductive system, such as pelvic inflammatory disease. *See* Pelvic inflammatory disease.

If you have abdominal pain, especially if it is continuous and becomes more severe, see a doctor promptly. You may need antibiotics for an infection, or other drugs or treatment.

Abdominal thrusts. *See* Heimlich maneuver.

Abnormal. The term means not within the usual (normal) range, but does not necessarily signify illness or disease. For example, a person may be abnormally tall or short, yet be a healthy person in every way.

Abnormality. An unusual condition of a body part, such as a birth defect or deformity; or a poorly or improperly functioning organ caused by an infection or disease; or a lab test result out of the normal range.

Abortion. The termination of a pregnancy during its early stages. An abortion may occur due to a mishap, or as the result of a hormonal disturbance or other abnormality (spontaneous abortion, miscarriage). An abortion may also be performed, using one of several methods. In the first trimester, these include vacuum curettage, dilation and curettage, or dilation and evacuation. A recently introduced procedure involves the use of an oral drug, RU-486. *See* RU-486.

An abortion may be performed in the second trimester (third to sixth month of pregnancy). A two-step procedure may be used. First laminaria (seaweed) is inserted to soften the cervix. The following day, the abortion is performed.

In the United States, legal abortions performed in licensed clinics are generally safe.

Complications of abortion: A person who has had an abortion should see a doctor promptly if she notices the following signs: fever, chills, muscle aches, fatigue, cramps and abdominal pain, heavy bleeding, a foul vaginal discharge, or a delay of six weeks or longer before the next menstrual period.

Abrasion. A scratch or scrape somewhere on the body, for example, the knee, that may bleed.

Abscess. A pus-filled area on the skin or inside the body; usually the result of an infection.

Abstinence. Not having sex.

Abuse. An act that causes physical or mental harm to another person. The various forms of abuse include child sexual abuse, physical, sexual, and verbal abuse. Excessive

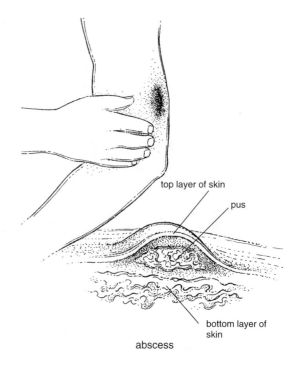

top layer of skin

pus

bottom layer of skin

abscess

use of alcohol, food, or drugs can be self-abuse.

Child sexual abuse: Touching, fondling, or sexually molesting a child.

Drug abuse: See Drug abuse.

Physical abuse: Hitting, slapping, or beating a person.

Sexual abuse: Touching or fondling another person's breasts, genital area, or other body parts against that person's will.

Verbal abuse: Using words to put down, demean, or attack another person.

Accutane. A drug used to treat acne. *See* Acne; Appendix B: Acne medications.

Achalasia. A relatively rare disorder of the nerves and muscles in the food tube (esophagus). Food does not pass normally to the stomach, but remains in the food tube or is regurgitated (comes back up). Treatment involves a procedure to stretch the muscles of the food tube or, sometimes, surgery.

Acne. A skin condition that often occurs during teenage years.

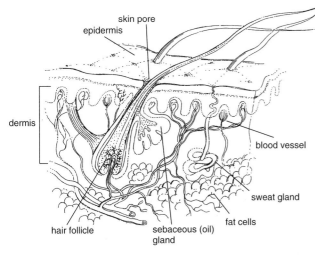

skin pore
epidermis
dermis
blood vessel
sweat gland
fat cells
hair follicle
sebaceous (oil) gland

How acne develops:
1. Oil glands secrete sebum that may block a hair follicle.
2. A plug forms over the skin pore, and sebum collects in the blocked follicle.
3. Bacteria infect the sebum, leading to inflammation.

Causes: Certain hormones (substances produced by glands) increase during the teen years. These hormones stimulate oil glands under the skin to produce extra oil, which plugs the small ducts that lead from the gland to the skin and causes inflammation (acne). You may be more likely to develop acne if your father or mother had acne during their teens. Acne occurs most often on the face, chest, or back in the form of pimples filled with pus or oil.

Misconceptions: Some teens believe that
* Acne improves with frequent, hard scrubbing
* Acne is caused, or made worse, by eating certain foods such as chocolate, fried foods, or nuts
* Acne is improved by exposure to sunlight
* Acne is incurable
  None of these beliefs are true.

If you overscrub, your skin will become irritated, and possibly crack and become infected.

There is no proof that eating chocolate or nuts causes or aggravates acne. However, some teens may be sensitive to iodine, which is found in shellfish and iodized table salt. They should therefore avoid these foods.

Extensive exposure to sunlight does not improve acne. It may make it worse and, over time, predispose to skin cancer.

The worst misconception is that acne is incurable. This causes unnecessary distress and unhappiness, and it is not true. It may be impossible to prevent acne, but it can almost always be greatly improved, and in many cases cleared up completely, with the help of a physician and effective medications.

Treatment: Over-the-counter medication or medication prescribed by a doctor. A healthful diet and lifestyle may also help. *See* Appendix B, Acne medications.

Acquired immunodeficiency syndrome (AIDS). *See* AIDS.

Acupuncture. A treatment method of Chinese origin, used widely in that country to control pain and alleviate many other conditions. With this technique, very fine needles are inserted at certain points in the body that are believed to control the path of energy in various directions. According to theory, this energy runs along a grid of nerve channels throughout the body. Pain and other symptoms may develop if the "nerve" channels are blocked; once they are reopened with acupuncture, the complaints are relieved.

Acute. Any symptom, disease, or other condition that arises suddenly. *See* Chronic.

ADD (Attention Deficit Disorder). A disorder in young children, with symptoms that may include a short attention span, impulsive behavior, and hyperactivity. The disorder is far more common in boys than in girls, and may continue throughout the teen years, and even into adulthood. The cause is unknown.

Treatment includes psychotherapy and

drugs; for example, antidepressants (imipramine), or psychostimulants such as methylphenidate (Ritalin).

Addiction. Dependency on the regular use of certain substances such as alcohol, tobacco, stimulants, narcotics, or other drugs. The effects of these substances on the body and nervous system are often so strong that addicts cannot carry out their daily activities without taking the drugs at regular intervals. Most addictive substances are harmful to the body, especially if taken over long periods of time. *See also* Appendix C, Street Drugs.

Adenoids. Lymph gland tissue located in the back of the throat behind the nose. When adenoids are enlarged as a result of infection, allergy, or for other reasons, breathing through the nose may be difficult. Snoring is often a symptom. In severe cases, surgery may be necessary.

Adolescence. The period in life that begins with puberty and ends with adulthood.

Aerobic exercise. A form of exercise that stimulates the heart, with a corresponding increase in the heart and breathing rate.

AIDS. A group of diseases and symptoms, all caused by a virus that weakens and destroys the immune system.

Cause: The human immunodeficiency virus (HIV).

How AIDS affects people: The AIDS syndrome affects people in different ways. Some persons infected with HIV stay apparently healthy for many years and show no symptoms of illness. Others develop one or more AIDS-related diseases, become very ill, and die.

HIV destroys the immune system, which fights off infections and diseases. As the immune system weakens, it allows harmful organisms to invade the body and set up infections.

Transmission of HIV infection: Through unprotected sexual contact between a healthy and an infected person. The infection is also transmitted by HIV-infected blood or other infected body fluids that enter a healthy person's bloodstream, either by way of a transfusion of infected blood or through a needle puncture. HIV infection may also be transmitted from an infected pregnant woman to her baby through exposure to the placenta or, later, through breast milk.

Detection of HIV infection: A blood test developed in 1985 determines the presence of HIV antibodies; a positive test indicates exposure to HIV, and probably HIV infection. The test is also used to check donor blood. HIV-infected blood is discarded. Blood donors are screened before giving blood, to ensure a safe blood supply for those who need to receive whole blood or one of its components. A newer test (PCR) can detect the presence of the virus in the blood. The antibody test is more commonly used. It can show positive results several weeks to several months after exposure.

Treatment: Various medications and other treatments slow down the progress of HIV infection and the development of AIDS. They include zidovudine (AZT), a newer class of drugs called protease inhibitors (saquinavir, indinavir, ritonavir), and others. To date, there is no treatment that produces a cure.

Many HIV-infected people develop AIDS within five to ten years. Researchers are working to develop more effective medications and a vaccine to protect people from this terrible illness. An HIV-infected pregnant woman who takes the drug zidovudine (AZT) before delivery and for a short period afterward can greatly reduce the risk that the baby will be infected. Newborns at risk of

HIV infection are also given AZT, to reduce the risk.

Special precautions: You can protect yourself against HIV infection in these ways:

- Be sexually responsible. HIV can be transmitted during sexual intercourse. Do not have sex with anyone whose sexual and health history you don't know. Say no to sex when you are not sure.
- Avoid alcohol and other drugs. These may impair judgment about sex and condom use.
- During sex, always use a latex condom that contains nonoxynol-9. Be sure to use condoms correctly. *See* Condom, female; Condom, male.
- Avoid contact with the blood and body fluids of any person who may be infected with HIV. Do not handle needles, knives, or other items that may carry the virus. If you are scratched or cut, the virus in infected blood or body fluid may infect you.

Alanon. An organization that helps people who are trying to cope with alcoholism in their families. Local chapters are listed in the telephone directory.

Alateen. An organization that helps teens cope with problems caused by alcoholism—either their own or that of a family member. Look up Alateen in your local telephone directory.

Alcohol. A substance in drinks such as wine, beer, or whiskey. Alcohol is dangerous when used often, or in large quantities.

Effects of alcohol: Alcohol can cause physical and mental damage. Alcohol impairs brain function and therefore coordination and judgment. It is particularly dangerous for people to drive after alcohol use. Frequent alcohol use can also cause damage to other organs, especially the liver. Excessive alcohol use may lead to the development of cancer in various organs. A pregnant woman who drinks even a small amount of alcohol may place her unborn baby at risk for damaged organs and other long-lasting, serious illnesses. *See also* Fetal alcohol syndrome.

Alcohol overdose. *See* Appendix C.

Alcoholics Anonymous (AA). An organization that helps people with alcohol problems overcome their addiction. Members meet several times a week, and sometimes every day, to discuss their drinking. They support each other as they learn to manage life and its problems without using alcohol. AA is listed in local telephone directories.

Allergic dermatitis. *See* Contact dermatitis.

Allergy. An adverse body reaction that occurs after a person is exposed to a substance to which he or she is unusually sensitive.

Substances that can cause allergic reactions include certain foods, drugs, and other substances such as cosmetics. Allergic reactions may occur after use of a substance or drug on the skin; ingesting it by mouth, by inhalation, or by injection. Exposure to animal venom, as in a bee sting or snake bite, may cause a dangerous allergic reaction in a person who is hypersensitive to the substance (having been exposed before).

Severity of reactions: Some people have more severe allergic reactions than others. For example, in a nonallergic person, a bee sting may cause only slight redness and swelling at the site of the sting, plus a little discomfort. A moderately allergic person may develop a larger swelling, more severe redness, and considerable discomfort. Minor allergic reactions may progress to severe ones after repeated exposures. A severely allergic person may develop life-threatening symptoms that

Allergic reactions may appear after exposure to an allergy-causing substance through

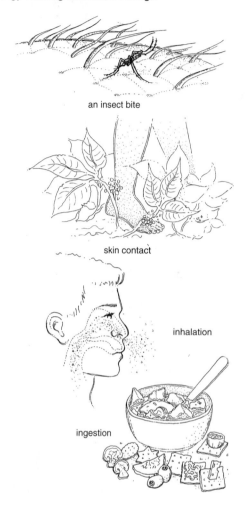

an insect bite

skin contact

inhalation

ingestion

require immediate emergency treatment. *See also* Anaphylaxis.

Treatment: An allergist (a doctor who specializes in treating people with allergic conditions) can provide treatment to reduce or eliminate allergic reactions, through medications or other techniques. *See also* Patch test; Skin tests.

Alopecia. *See* Hair loss.

Alternative medicine. A variety of treatment methods that may be different from those commonly used in general medical practice. Some people prefer approaches of alternative medicine over standard medical treatments because they believe alternative medical treatment is more effective, or because regular medical treatment has not helped with a problem. Other people prefer alternative medicine because they believe it is just as effective, but less expensive and causes fewer side effects.

In recent years, alternative medicine has received considerable attention. Many doctors believe that studies should be conducted to test the value of various alternative treatment techniques, so that those shown to be beneficial in carefully controlled scientific studies can be used along with other medical treatments. *See also* Acupuncture; Homeopathy; Chiropractic; Herbalism; Naturopathy; Spiritual healing; Holistic health care; Biofeedback.

Amenorrhea. Absence of menstrual periods. Primary amenorrhea exists when a teenage girl (over sixteen) has never had a menstrual period. Secondary amenorrhea occurs when a teenage girl starts having regular periods, then skips her period for a month or more at a time.

Amniocentesis. Insertion of a needle into the amniotic sac that surrounds the fetus in a pregnant woman's uterus, to withdraw (amniotic) fluid from the sac for examination. This procedure is usually performed when a woman is fifteen to seventeen weeks pregnant. Examination of the fluid may show abnormalities or disease of the fetus. Cells may be examined to determine the sex of the fetus.

Amnion. The fluid-filled sac that surrounds and protects the fetus in the mother's womb (uterus) during pregnancy.

Amniotic fluid. Fluid in the amniotic sac that cushions and protects the growing fetus inside the mother's womb during pregnancy.

Anabolic steroids. Synthetic hormones, sometimes used illegally by athletes to build muscle strength. These hormones are very dangerous and can cause liver disease, cancer, infertility (inability to have a child), impotence (inability to have an erection), and other illnesses. These conditions may continue even after the hormones are stopped. *See also* Steroids.

Analgesic. A drug that relieves pain. *See also* Appendix B: Medications and Their Use.

Anaphylaxis, Anaphylactic shock. A severe allergic reaction that may be fatal if it is not treated immediately with medication and other procedures. *See also* Allergy.

Androgen. A male sex hormone that produces male characteristics, including mature male sex organs, a deep voice, and a beard.

Anemia. A condition in which there are too few red blood cells and too little hemoglobin in the blood to nourish body tissues. Anemia in teens is often caused by iron deficiency. Iron is essential in forming hemoglobin, the pigment in red blood cells that carries oxygen to nourish body tissues. With a shortage of iron in the blood, too few red blood cells are available to carry enough oxygen for the body's needs, or the existing blood cells may be too small.

Teens may develop iron deficiency as a result of rapid growth, poor eating habits, and (in girls) the onset of menstrual periods. Other teens have anemia due to genetic causes or blood diseases such as sickle-cell disease or thalassemia.

Anesthesia. A process used to prevent pain during surgery and certain other painful diagnostic or treatment procedures. There are two main types of anesthesia: general anesthesia and local anesthesia. General anesthesia is usually given during major surgery by an anesthesiologist, a medical specialist who administers certain drugs by way of inhalation or injection. The patient loses consciousness and awakes only after the operation is completed.

Local anesthesia is usually given for a shorter treatment or diagnostic procedure. Drugs are administered by direct (topical) application to the operative area, or by injection.

Aneurysm. A dilated (distended) area in some portion of the wall of an artery, caused by weakness or disease. Most often, an aneurysm is found in an artery in the brain, heart, or abdomen. An aneurysm may be small, then become larger as disease and the pressure of blood further damage and thin out the arterial wall. Without treatment, an aneurysm may burst, causing fatal bleeding unless surgery is done immediately, to stop the bleeding and repair the damaged artery.

Symptoms depend on the aneurysm's size and location. If it is in the brain and bursts, symptoms may include intense headache, vision problems, and loss of consciousness. Symptoms of an abdominal aorta aneurysm depend on the location. In the abdomen, a small aneurysm may cause no symptoms for some time; as it grows larger, it may press on an organ and cause discomfort. A doctor may hear sounds through the stethoscope that indicate the presence of an aneurysm. An aneurysm located higher up in a person's chest may cause chest pain (making the person fear he or she is having a heart attack), hoarseness, or difficulty in swallowing.

An aneurysm is a dangerous, potentially fatal problem. Any person who suddenly has a severe headache, or develops pain or a throbbing lump somewhere in the abdomen, needs immediate medical attention.

Angel dust (PCP). A potent substance (chemical name: phencyclidine) used illegally by some drug abusers. Angel dust is a dangerous street drug usually sold in powder form.

When PCP is sprinkled on tobacco, smoked and inhaled, or injected, it at first provides a feeling of well-being. But after a short time, the user feels anxious and depressed. After taking larger amounts of PCP, other physical symptoms appear. They include joint pain and a state of inertia called catatonia in which the person becomes stiff and does not react to stimuli. The user may also become hyperactive, with muscles jerking out of control and with the eyes moving in an abnormal way. Very large amounts of the substance may cause loss of consciousness, seizures, high blood pressure, and death.

Angiogram. A type of X ray to determine a problem in one or more of the major blood vessels. Such problems include a blockage, or aneurysm (a weakening of a blood vessel wall). During the angiogram, a type of dye is injected into a vein or artery, making the blood vessel more easily visible on the X ray.

Angioplasty. A surgical procedure to reduce fatty deposits that block the flow of blood from major blood vessels, such as the arteries in the heart.

Anonymous. Unidentified. For example, a person who takes a blood test anonymously cannot be identified.

Anorexia nervosa. A condition, most often seen in teenage girls, and also in young women and occasionally in boys, in which the teen starves herself or himself, due to a distorted self-image and excessive fear of obesity.

  Symptoms: Poor or no appetite; inability to maintain normal body weight; dangerous, often life-threatening weight loss; in girls menstruation may stop. Although often close to starvation, the anorexic person believes that nothing is wrong

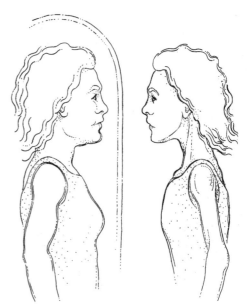

The anorexic person sees herself as fat, while to others, she is gaunt and bony.

and that she is eating an adequate amount of food. While visibly too thin, she is convinced that she is overweight.

  Treatment: Without specialized treatment, including psychological counseling and dietary therapy, the anorexic person may starve to death. In severe cases, treatment may require hospitalization, intravenous feeding, and psychiatric treatment.

Antepartum. The period of time before a baby is born.

Antibiotic. A substance or drug that can kill microorganisms harmful to the human body. Antibiotics are used to treat many different types of infections.

Antibody. A protein blood factor that develops when a foreign body (antigen) invades the body. The antibody fights off infections. *See also* Antigen.

Antibody test. A test to see if antibodies to certain antigens are present in the blood. If the antibody to an infectious agent is found, the doctor knows the patient has been exposed to that infection, and starts treatment, if needed.

Antifungals. Medications used to treat fungal infections. *See* Appendix B: Medications and Their Use.

Antigen. A foreign substance introduced into the body that causes antibodies to develop to fight it. Sometimes the body's immune system mistakes normal body cells or protein for a foreign substance and attacks, causing illness. An antigen may be a component of a virus or a bacterium. *See also* Antibody; Immune system.

Antigen test. A test to show whether a particular antigen is present in the blood. If an antigen is found, the infection or disease causing it to be present can be identified, and specific treatment given.

Antiviral. Word used to describe a substance or medication that fights a virus.

Anus. The lowest portion, about 1 inch to $1^1/2$ inches long, of the rectum. The anus is the end portion of the intestinal tract—the digestive tube that begins at the mouth. *See* Digestive system.

Anxiety. Fearfulness or apprehension. Many teens and other people feel anxious at certain times, for example, before taking an exam, meeting a new date, or during an illness. An anxious person may have sweaty hands, a fast pulse, and rapid respirations. This type of anxiety usually stops once the critical situation ends.

A person who feels anxious much of the time, and cannot give a reason for it, should consult a psychotherapist. This mental health professional provides counseling and other treatment as needed.

Aphasia. Difficulty in speaking or inability to speak caused by damage to the brain's language center. Speech therapy may relieve this problem to an extent.

Aphrodisiac. A substance that is supposed to stimulate or increase sexual desire.

Appendectomy. Surgical removal of the appendix, which may be necessary if it becomes inflamed. *See* Appendix.

Appendix. A worm-shaped intestinal structure 3 to 4 inches long that is attached to the cecum, the first part of the large bowel.

Arrhythmia. Irregularity of the heartbeat. This may be harmless and temporary, as when a person is excited or nervous, or it may indicate a heart problem. *See* Palpitation.

Arthritis. An inflammatory condition of the joints, such as the knuckles, elbows, knees, or shoulders.

Causes: Arthritis may be caused by an infection such as gonorrhea, by injury to the joints, or by an autoimmune disease such as systemic lupus erythematosus (SLE), juvenile rheumatoid arthritis (JRA), or rheumatoid arthritis (RA).

Symptoms: Pain, redness, swelling, fluid accumulation, and poor mobility of the affected joints.

Treatment: Depends on the type of arthritis diagnosed. It may include rest, anti-inflammatory drugs, antibiotics, and physical therapy.

See also Rheumatoid arthritis; Juvenile rheumatoid arthritis.

Arthrocentesis. Aspiration (taking fluid from a joint) to remove excess fluid built up during injury or disease.

Arthroscopy. A procedure in which a doctor inserts a small tube fitted with a light into a joint to look for possible injury. Surgical instruments may then be passed through the tube to correct a problem. This type of surgery has two advantages: it causes only a tiny wound, which allows for a quick recovery, and it leaves a very small scar.

Artificial insemination. A medical procedure to impregnate a woman. A doctor takes sperm collected from the husband or from a donor and injects it into the woman's cervix (entrance to the womb). The procedure is performed in the middle of the menstrual cycle, when the woman's egg is on its way to the uterus or is already in the uterus. The egg can then be fertilized by the injected sperm to start a pregnancy.

Artificial respiration. Physically helping a person who is having trouble breathing. *See also* Appendix F: First Aid, Rescue breathing; Cardiopulmonary resuscitation.

Asexual. The absence of sexual identity or sexual feelings.

Aspirate (n). The fluid or tissue withdrawn by a doctor from somewhere inside the body.

Aspirate (v). To draw fluid from somewhere inside the body, for diagnostic or treatment purposes. A doctor may aspirate some fluid from the lungs (thoracentesis), to diagnose a problem in that area. Or, a doctor may aspirate fluid from a swollen and inflamed knee, to relieve pain and pressure inside the knee joint.

Aspiration. A procedure done for diagnostic or treatment purposes, in which some fluid or tissue is withdrawn from some part of the body.

Asthma. A condition marked by wheezing and difficulty in breathing.
  Causes: Asthma is caused by swelling or spasms of the bronchial tube (a part of the respiratory tract) and by production of thick mucus that blocks or decreases the air reaching the lungs. An asthma attack may be triggered by fatigue, allergy, emotional stress, or exposure to toxic fumes or cold air. Other causes may not yet be known.
  Symptom: Wheezing or difficulty in breathing.
  Treatments for asthma include:
  • Oral medications: Bronchodilators such as Alupent, Ventolin, and theophylline. Steroid drugs such as prednisone, which acts as an anti-inflammatory agent and reduces swelling.
  • Inhalers: Anti-inflammatory agents such as Intal, and steroid drugs such as Azmacort or Vanceril. Bronchodilators such as Alupent and Ventolin.
  See also Appendix B, Asthma medications.

Astigmatism. *See* Eye disorders.

Atacques. A condition that may follow great stress or emotional problems. An affected person may seem "out of it" for a short while, or may have movements similar to those of a seizure.

Athlete's foot. A fungal infection that usually affects the spaces between the toes. *See also* Fungal infection.

Attention deficit disorder. *See* ADD.

Audiogram. A hearing test that measures eardrum vibrations and detects fluid that may be trapped behind the eardrum, which may interfere with hearing. *See also* Deafness.

Autoimmune. This term refers to the body's use of antibodies to some of its own tissues, causing damage. As a result, certain diseases, called autoimmune diseases, may develop. These include rheumatoid arthritis and lupus erythematosus. *See also* Rheumatoid arthritis, Lupus erythematosus.

Autoimmune disorder. A condition in which the body makes antibodies that attack its own tissues and cause a variety of diseases. *See also* Autoimmune.

Asthma
Pollen, dust, smoke, or other irritants enter the nose or mouth and cause swelling of the air passages (bronchi, bronchioles).

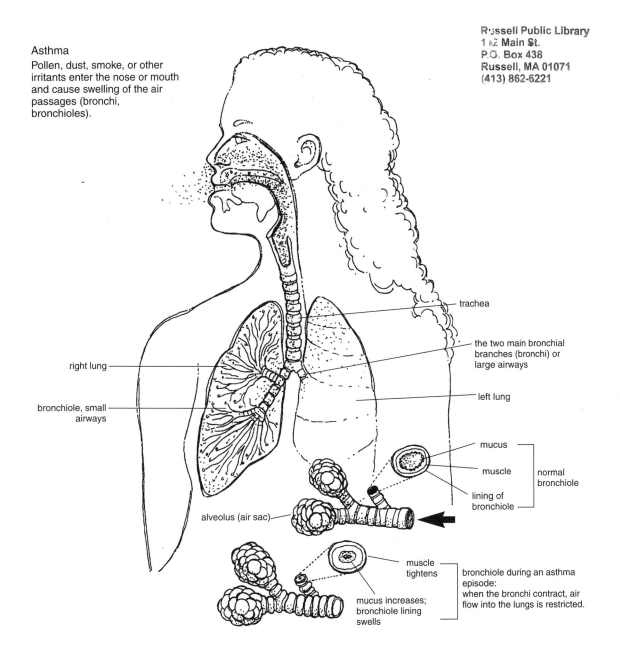

trachea

the two main bronchial branches (bronchi) or large airways

right lung

left lung

bronchiole, small airways

mucus

muscle

normal bronchiole

lining of bronchiole

alveolus (air sac)

muscle tightens

bronchiole during an asthma episode:
when the bronchi contract, air flow into the lungs is restricted.

mucus increases; bronchiole lining swells

B

Bacilli. Bacteria that resemble short rods when seen under a microscope. They may cause serious illnesses such as whooping cough, dysentery, and typhoid fever.

***Bacillus Calmette Guérin* (BCG).** A weak strain of the organism that causes tuberculosis, used as a vaccine to prevent or lessen the chance of contracting tuberculosis. (Not routinely used in the United States.)

Bacteria. Microscopic, one-celled germs (microbes) that exist in many different shapes. Bacteria live everywhere: in water, soil, air, and in living organisms. Some are useful, such as those that aid in the production of plant foods. Others are harmful and cause many different infections, including strep throat and tuberculosis.

Bad breath (halitosis). An unpleasant odor or taste in the mouth. Temporary bad breath may be caused by eating onions, garlic, or other foods with a strong flavor or odor. Longer lasting bad breath may signal infection of the gums, teeth, tonsils, or sinuses. Treatment of the infection will clear up the bad breath. Poorly digested foods (for example, milk and other dairy products are difficult for some people to digest), can cause bad breath when unpleasant gases or odors are released through the mouth. Eliminating these foods usually solves the problem.

Balding. *See* Hair loss.

Barrier contraceptive. *See* Contraceptive.

Bartholin's glands. Glands located on the vaginal lips (vulva). The openings of these glands may become clogged due to infection or inflammation, causing a painful fluid-filled swelling (cyst). Surgery may be needed to remove the cyst and clear up the infection.

Bedwetting. *See* Enuresis.

Benign. A condition or disease that, although abnormal, is not life-threatening and can be treated and cured in most instances.

Bestiality. *See* Sodomy.

Bile. A yellow fluid secreted by the liver that flows into the intestinal tract (the duodenum), where it aids in the digestion of fatty foods.

Bilirubin. Bile pigment.

Binge, binge eating. An episode of excessive, out-of-control eating or drinking. Binge drinkers may consume eight to ten drinks or more at one time. Binge eaters may eat an enormous amount of food in a short time. Binge eating may be followed by self-induced vomiting, or purging. *See also* Bulimia.

Biofeedback. A method of learning to control certain body processes—such as blood pressure, temperature, heart rate—and body reactions, and thereby reduce the effects of stress on the body. Electronic sensors attached to a person's body measure its responses. The feedback of information from the sensors helps the person learn, through practice, how to relax and regulate the body's reactions. Biofeedback therapy is used to help patients control stress, and in treatment of headaches, muscle spasms, and high blood pressure.

Biopsy. The surgical removal of a small piece of tissue for laboratory examination. Health care professionals use the laboratory report to make or confirm a diagnosis.

Bipolar disorder (manic depression). A mental disease that causes wide mood swings. A person with bipolar disorder may be deeply depressed for some time, then switch to a period of mania.

During the depressed period, the person with bipolar disorder may withdraw from most normal activities and friends and family, and speak very little, sleep a great deal, and feel that life is not worth living. *See also* Depression.

During the manic period, the person with bipolar disorder becomes overactive, sleeps only a short time at night, often has an increased sex drive, and may spend, or want to spend, huge amounts of money. The manic person may be elated (laughing, dancing, talking too much), or may believe he or she is a very important person (a king, queen, religious figure, president, a great authority or genius), or uniquely gifted. Often, these manic or depressive periods occur in cycles, alternating with periods of normal life, that vary from short to long. *See also* Mania.

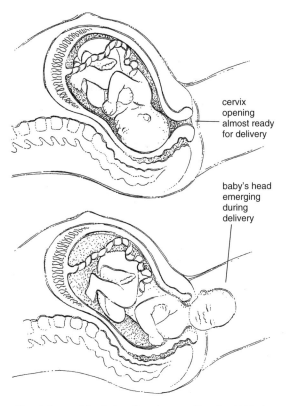

cervix opening almost ready for delivery

baby's head emerging during delivery

The delivery of the baby after nine months of pregnancy.

Birth. Delivery of a baby at the end of a pregnancy.

Birth control. Prevention of pregnancy by one of several methods available to both women and men.

Least effective methods:

For men: Withdrawal of the penis before ejaculation.

For women: Rhythm method; douching after sexual intercourse.

Most effective methods:

For men: condom; vasectomy.

For women: Diaphragm; cervical cap; female condom; contraceptive foam or jelly; vaginal suppositories; intrauterine device (IUD); the birth control pill; Depo-Provera, a hormone injected every three months; Norplant, a hormone implanted in a woman's arm to protect against pregnancy for up to five years.

See also the individual entries listed above; Morning-after pill; Oral contraceptive.

Birth control pill. A pill containing one or more hormones, taken regularly to prevent pregnancy. There are two main types.

Birth control pill, monophasic: A pill taken every day that releases equal amounts of the hormones estrogen and progesterone during the twenty-one days of the menstrual cycle, and no hormones during the last seven days of the cycle.

Birth control pill, triphasic: A pill taken every day that contains the hormones estrogen and progesterone. The dosage of estrogen stays constant for three weeks. The dosage of progesterone is increased somewhat, but only during the second week of the cycle. *See also* Contraceptive device, Morning-after pill, Oral contraceptive.

Birth defect. Abnormality of a body structure, portion, or system found at birth. A birth defect may be inherited, or develop during pregnancy or the birth process.

Birthmark (nevus, freckle, mole). An abnormal portion of overgrown skin, round or oval in shape, that contains color (pigment) or extra blood vessels. A birthmark may appear on the head or elsewhere on the body, at birth or shortly afterward.

Depending on the size and content of the birthmark, it may disappear, or require no treatment. Others, if unsightly, may be treated with steroid medication. Still others may be treated by laser therapy or surgery.

Any birthmark that changes in size, shape, or color needs to be examined by a skin doctor (dermatologist), to determine if a potentially dangerous skin condition such as skin cancer is beginning to develop. Treated early, skin cancer can be cured easily.

Bisexual. An individual who is sexually attracted both to males and to females. While many adolescents experiment sexually with other teens of the same sex as well as the opposite sex; most become heterosexual as they mature. Some teens remain bisexual and some may become exlusively homosexual.

Blackhead. *See* Comedone.

Bladder, urinary. The portion of the urinary tract that stores urine until it is eliminated from (has passed out of) the body. *See illustration* The Human Body.

Blindness (vision loss). Inability to see with one or both eyes. Vision loss occurs as a result of many different causes. It may be apparent at birth, caused by disease or infection contracted during pregnancy. A person may also become blind as a result of:
- Severe vitamin A deficiency
- Excessive pressure in the eye (glaucoma)
- Certain illnesses such as nervous system disease or undiagnosed, untreated diabetes

Blister. A sac of clear fluid or blood that develops under the skin's surface following friction or a crush injury. The skin covering the blister serves as a natural bandage; it should not be broken or removed while it is intact. *See also* Appendix F: First Aid, Blisters.

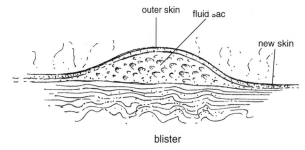

blister

Blood. Fluid that circulates through the body to nourish tissues, remove materials no longer needed, and regulate body temperature to some extent. Fresh (oxygenated) blood is pumped from the heart through the arteries to every part of the body, with nourishment (digested food, oxygen, and other essential substances) for all the body's tissues.

Veins return used (oxygen-depleted) blood to the lungs, which remove the waste gas, carbon dioxide. The blood then picks up new oxygen, returns to the heart, and is pumped back out into the body. A healthy person's body contains from three to six quarts of blood, and a healthy heart pumps about 1,250 gallons of blood per day. This is essential, for tissues cut off from a continuous blood supply will die within a few minutes.

Blood helps regulate body temperature. Blood vessels dilate to bring warm blood to the surface of the body (under the skin), where it is cooled on a warm day. If the outside temperature is cold, the blood vessels contract, preventing warm blood from reaching the surface of the body, and thus keeping the body warm.

Blood consists of many different parts (components): *Plasma* is the clear liquid portion (over 55 percent) of blood. Plasma is 92 percent water. It contains a protein (fibrinogen) that allows blood to clot when the skin is cut; and other substances, produced by the lymph glands, that help the body fight infection. Plasma carries enzymes, hormones, vitamins, salts, and still other substances needed by the body to function effectively.

Red blood cells, *White blood cells*, and *Platelets* are the solid constituents in blood.

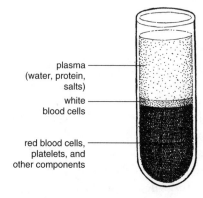

plasma (water, protein, salts)

white blood cells

red blood cells, platelets, and other components

blood components

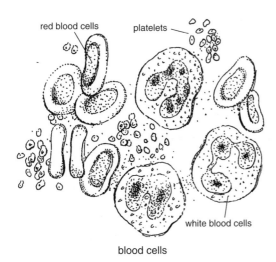

red blood cells   platelets

white blood cells

blood cells

Red blood cells and platelets are produced by the bone marrow. Red blood cells contain hemoglobin, which carries oxygen, and accounts for the red color of blood. Some of the white blood cells also originate in the bone marrow, and others are produced by the lymph glands. White blood cells help the body fight infections. Platelets help the blood to clot after an injury.

Blood pressure (BP). The pressure exerted by circulating blood against the walls of the blood vessels. *See* Hypertension.

Blood transfusion. *See* Transfusion.

Blue balls (stone ache). Some teenage boys mistakenly believe that their testicles will turn blue if they don't ejaculate after having an erection. This concern is unfounded. No temporary or permanent harm occurs if a male does not ejaculate after an erection.

Body mass index (BMI). A formula based on height, weight, and sex used to calculate the normal ranges of body weight.

To calculate your BMI, use this formula:

$$\frac{\text{weight in kilograms (kg)}}{\text{height in meters, squared (m}^2)}$$

Example: If your weight is 45 kg (100 pounds), and your height is 1.52 m (60 inches), your BMI is

$$\frac{45 \text{ kg}}{(1.52)^2 = 2.31} = \text{BMI of } 19.48$$

The normal BMI range is from 20 to 25.

Body piercing. *See* Piercing, body

Bone marrow aspiration. A test of red blood cells, white blood cells, and platelets—the major components of blood. A needle is inserted into the core (marrow) of a bony area to obtain a tissue sample. This important test is used in the diagnosis of diseases such as leukemia (a cancer of the white blood cells) and certain serious infections.

In infants and small children, and sometimes in adults, the bone marrow sample (bone marrow biopsy) is drawn from the breastbone; in older children, teens, and most adults, it is drawn from the crest of the hip.

Bone scan. *See* Radionuclide scan.

Bowel. The portion of the intestinal tract that runs from the lower end of the stomach to the rectum. Its functions include the digestion of food, reabsorption of fluids, and the elimination of waste. *See also* Digestive system.

Braces, dental. Wire supports to adjust poorly positioned teeth that interfere with chewing and sometimes with the appearance. Braces are prescribed and applied by an orthodontist, a dentist who specializes in correcting the bite and the position of the teeth.

Breakthrough bleeding. A mild to moderate degree of bleeding experienced by some young women when they start to use birth control pills. Breakthrough bleeding may occur several days (or weeks) before the true menstrual period is due to start. This bleeding is not harmful and does not indicate a health problem. It usually stops once the body adjusts to the pills. Breakthrough bleeding may also occur if a woman forgets to take her daily dose. This is remedied by doubling up—that is, by taking two pills—the next day.

Breast augmentation. The surgical enlargement of the breasts of young women who feel their breasts are too small. Surgeons implant a sac filled with gel or saline in each breast. The long-term safety of these implants is not certain, and some problems have been reported.

Breast development. One of the earliest signs of physical maturation in girls. Breast development continues through the teen years until the breasts reach adult size. All girls experience breast changes during puberty, but some girls' breasts develop more quickly than others.

Genetic factors may determine breast size, and some girls develop larger breasts than other girls. Many girls have one breast that is different from the other, either in size or shape. This is normal.

Some boys develop enlarged breasts—a condition called gynecomastia—as they mature. As a boy gets older, the breasts usually diminish in size. If not, the excessive breast tissue can be removed surgically.

Breast discharge. Fluid coming from the nipples. A nonpregnant, healthy teenager has no nipple discharge. If a girl does have nipple discharge, she should consult a doctor. The discharge may be unimportant if it appears after stimulation or irritation. However, it may indicate a glandular problem of the thyroid, situated in the neck, or of the pituitary gland, located in the brain, that requires treatment. Certain medications or drugs may cause a nipple discharge. *See also* Galactorrhea.

Breast reduction. A surgical procedure to reduce a woman's excessively large breasts.

Some girls or women with very large breasts experience back and chest pain. Others feel uncomfortable about the size of their breasts. A surgeon may perform an operation (reduction mammoplasty) to decrease the size of the breasts.

Breast self-examination. A procedure mature females should perform monthly to detect changes in the breasts that may require medical attention. The best time to perform the exam is just after the menstrual period. In many women, the breasts become larger a few days before their period. This is a normal occurrence and no cause for concern.

Significant changes include a lump or a thickening in the breasts, a discharge from the nipples, and changes in the color of the skin surrounding the nipples. Lumps and other changes may be benign and temporary, or they may require treatment.

Bronchodilation. The widening, or opening, of the breathing passages, usually achieved by medication. *See also* Asthma.

Bronchoscopy. Examination of the bronchi (breathing tubes that lead to the lungs), to check for disease or a foreign body. *See also* Endoscopy.

Bronchospasm. The tightening of the breathing tubes, causing a respiratory problem. The breathing passages in the lungs (bronchi and bronchioles) are lined with mucous glands and strands of muscle tissue and nerves.

Certain chemicals, gases, and other agents can activate nerves in the respiratory system. The muscles constrict, or tighten up (go into spasms), or cause mucous secretions. These spasms narrow the breathing passageways, cause wheezing, and result in breathing difficulties. Medication is available to activate other nerves and muscles that will stimulate the breathing tubes to reopen (bronchodila-

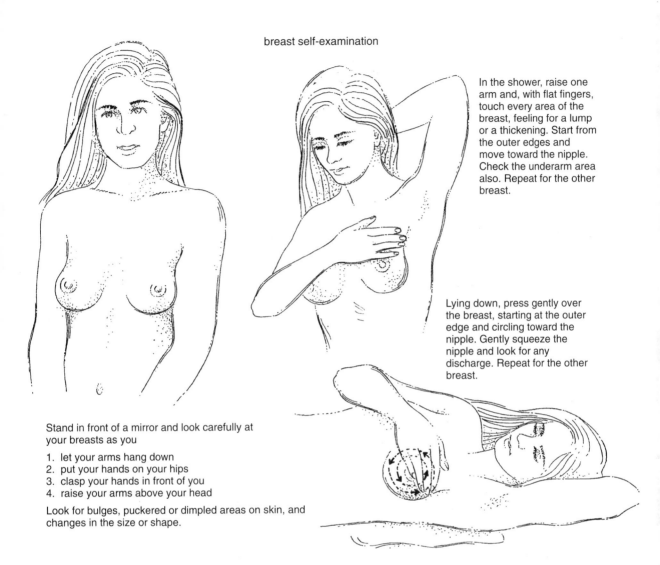

breast self-examination

In the shower, raise one arm and, with flat fingers, touch every area of the breast, feeling for a lump or a thickening. Start from the outer edges and move toward the nipple. Check the underarm area also. Repeat for the other breast.

Lying down, press gently over the breast, starting at the outer edge and circling toward the nipple. Gently squeeze the nipple and look for any discharge. Repeat for the other breast.

Stand in front of a mirror and look carefully at your breasts as you

1. let your arms hang down
2. put your hands on your hips
3. clasp your hands in front of you
4. raise your arms above your head

Look for bulges, puckered or dimpled areas on skin, and changes in the size or shape.

tion). *See also* Asthma; Appendix B, Asthma medications.

Bruise. An injury to the skin from a fall or blow may cause bleeding into the tissues below the skin, producing a reddish-blue discolored area and, sometimes, pain and swelling, which may last for several weeks. *See also* Appendix F: First Aid, Bruises.

Bulimia. An eating disorder primarily seen in girls and young women who eat excessive amounts of food, either occasionally or over a period of time. A person with bulimia often induces vomiting after overeating. Excessive eating is very difficult to stop. Professional counseling is essential, and hospitalization may be needed for successful treatment. *See also* Binge.

Bunion. An inflammation and tenderness of the big toe's bursa, a fluid-filled shock absorber. This condition is usually caused by wearing tight shoes over a long period. Without treatment, the big toe becomes twisted, and a large, painful knot develops on the instep. Surgery can correct this condition.

Burn. An injury of the skin or deeper tissues, caused by heat, a chemical, electricity, or radiation. Burns are classified by degree. In a first degree burn, the skin turns red; there are no blisters. Only the top layer of skin (epidermis) is affected. In a second degree burn, the skin turns very red and blisters form on its surface. In a third degree burn, the injury extends to the dermis (layer beneath the epidermis). Nerve endings in the dermis may be burned, thus producing less pain than in a more superficial burn.

All but superficial burns need immediate medical attention, to prevent complications such as infection, shock, and permanent tissue damage. *See also* Appendix F: First Aid, Burns.

Burner. *See* Stinger.

C

Cancer. A disease in which certain cells in the body multiply in a disorderly fashion and become increasingly abnormal. As these abnormal cells multiply, they crowd out normal cells and interfere with the normal functioning of the affected organ or body part.

There are many different types of cancer. Each destroys normal body tissues or systems. Successful treatments using surgery, radiation, and chemotherapy have been developed for various cancers. Early diagnosis and prompt treatment offer the best chance for a cure or for arresting the spread of the cancer.

To prevent cancer
- Don't smoke or chew tobacco
- Follow a low-fat, healthy diet, with plenty of fruits, vegetables, and whole-grain products
- Keep your weight at a healthy level
- Avoid alcohol use
- Use a sunscreen to protect your skin
- Take precautions to avoid sexually transmitted diseases. Practice Safer Sex

---

Warning signs of cancer
- A mole that grows larger, changes in shape or color, itches or bleeds
- Lumps or swellings
- Frequent indigestion
- Lingering hoarseness
- Lingering cough, coughing up blood
- Sores that do not heal
- Blood in the stool or urine
- Vaginal bleeding between menstrual periods

Candidiasis. A yeast infection.

Cause: A yeastlike organism called *Candida*, which attacks the genitals, and occasionally the skin, the nails, the mucous membranes of the mouth, and the respiratory tract.

Symptoms in men: Itching or pain; redness on the tip, sides, and foreskin of the penis.

Symptoms in women: Sticky, thick, white vaginal discharge; red, scaly appearance of the external genitals.

Other symptoms in men and women: White patches in the mouth or on the tongue; difficulty in swallowing.

Transmission:
- Certain medications, including antibiotics and some over-the-counter drugs, kill organisms that normally keep yeast cells under control. Without these organisms, yeast cells can multiply and cause infection
- Occasionally, but less often, by sexual intercourse with an infected partner
- A damaged immune system. Those who have HIV infection or AIDS may develop candidiasis because their immune system is too weak to fight off infection

Treatment: Effective medications are available that cure candidiasis. *See* Appendix B, Antifungal medications.

Special precautions: Avoid having sex with an infected person. If you are taking antibiotic medication, the doctor may prescribe an antiyeast medication as a preventive measure. Eating yogurt that contains acidophilus may also help prevent a yeast infection.

Carbohydrates (CHO). Chemical compounds that include various types of sugar and starch. Carbohydrates are a major source of energy.

Cardiac arrest. The stopping of the heartbeat. Death will occur unless measures are taken to restart the heart within a few minutes. A heart may stop spontaneously in a very aged person, or in someone with heart disease. Cardiac arrest may occur in younger people as a result of disease, an operation, or an overdose of prescribed medication or street drugs.

Various procedures are used to reverse cardiac arrest. The process is known as cardiac resuscitation and it can be carried out manually or with a defibrillator, a machine that uses electricity to shock the heart into beating again. This must be done within a few minutes of the arrest or the person will die. *See also* Appendix F: First Aid.

Cardiopulmonary resuscitation (CPR). A life-saving procedure used to restart the heart and respirations if a person's heart and breathing have slowed or stopped (cardiorespiratory arrest) due to injury or illness. CPR must be used promptly to prevent damage to the brain and other organs. *See also* Cardiac arrest; Appendix F: First Aid.

Cartilage. A semihard tissue that covers bone and joint surfaces. Cartilage acts as a shock absorber: it prevents friction between bones and joints, allowing them to function smoothly.

Casual contact. Social activity in which HIV or sexually transmitted diseases cannot be spread by an infected person. Sitting next to a person, having dinner together, working alongside each other, and hugging are all casual contacts.

CAT scan. *See* CT scan.

Cat scratch disease (fever). A mild infection caused by bacilli transmitted in scratches from a cat that carries the germs. A red, crusted papule develops at the site of the scratch in three to ten days. Swollen lymph nodes may develop in the area and the person may develop fever, headache, and feelings of general illness. Treatment consists of application of warm compresses, and a pain reliever, if necessary. In more severe cases, antibiotics may be needed.

Catheter. A thin, flexible tube made of rubber, plastic, or metal, used to:
- Remove body fluids (urine), for diagnostic purposes or if a person cannot urinate
- Diagnose certain illnesses, such as heart disease (via cardiac catheterization)
- Inject fluids and other substances intravenously or by other means to provide medications and food, if a person is unable to eat normally

Cauterization. Use of an instrument to burn abnormal or excessive tissues by means of electric current, a chemical substance such as silver nitrate, or heat. May also be used to stop bleeding in certain cases.

Cavities. *See* Dental caries.

CD4 cell. A white blood cell (T cell) in the immune system that helps the body to fight infection. Used by physicians as a marker of how significantly HIV infection has affected the immune system. Low CD4 counts indicate higher risk of opportunistic infections. *See also* Immune system; T cell.

Cecum. The first section of the large bowel, located in the right lower abdomen. *See* Digestive system.

Celibacy. Voluntary avoidance of sexual intercourse.

Centers for Disease Control and Prevention (CDC). A U.S. government agency that is responsible for watching over and preserving the health of the American people. The scientists, doctors, and other employees of the CDC work to prevent and control the spread of many diseases and dangerous infections in several ways:

- They track and study infections and diseases reported by doctors, clinics, and hospitals
- They require doctors to report certain infectious diseases such as gonorrhea and syphilis
- They issue regulations designed to stop the spread of disease and infection
- They conduct research and educational programs to discover treatments that will improve the health of the American people
- They provide information and recommendations for citizens planning foreign travel

Cerebral palsy (CP). A condition caused by damage to a baby's brain before, during, or after birth. Children with cerebral palsy have problems with muscle control, and may experience involuntary muscle movements or spasms of the face, neck, arms, and legs. Cerebral palsy ranges from mild and barely noticeable to severe, allowing little or no control of physical function.

Treatment for CP varies according to severity. Muscle spasms may respond to physical therapy and medication. Surgery is sometimes used to correct disabilities.

Cerebrospinal fluid (CSF). *See* Spinal fluid.

Cerumen. Wax in the ear canal.

Cervical cap. A soft rubber contraceptive device that fits closely over a woman's cervix (entrance to the womb). The cervical cap is smaller than a diaphragm and can be left in place for several days. It is prescribed by a

How to insert a cervical cap

the cervical cap

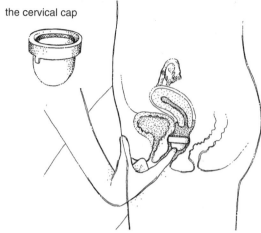

The cap is inserted gently into the vagina. The index finger is used to move the cap toward the cervix.

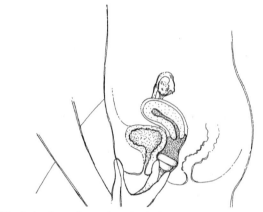

The index finger is used to check the position of the cap.

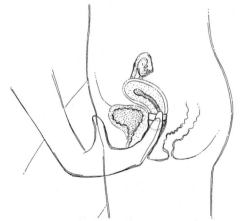

When in position, the cervical cap fits closely over the cervix and stays in place through suction.

doctor or other health professional. *See also* Contraception.

Cervix. The entrance to the womb (uterus). *See also* Reproductive system, female.

Cesarean section. A surgical procedure to deliver a baby through an incision in the mother's abdomen. A cesarean section is performed when the baby cannot be delivered safely through the mother's vagina. The fetus may show signs of serious illness and need medical treatment. Or, the mother may be ill and early delivery is necessary to save her life. In some women, the birth canal is too small to allow safe passage of the baby, and an abdominal delivery is needed. A woman who has a cesarean section may be able to deliver a subsequent baby in a normal labor and delivery procedure.

CFS. *See* Chronic fatigue syndrome.

Chancre. A small, round, raw-looking sore; the first sign of syphilis, a sexually transmitted disease. The chancre develops in the genital area of a healthy person after intercourse with an infected sexual partner. It is usually painless. *See also* Syphilis.

Chancroid. A sexually transmitted disease.
Cause: The organism *Hemophilus ducreyi.*
Symptoms: Painful sores in the genital area that develop into one or more larger, deep ulcers. The lymph glands near the genital area may become swollen and infected. Scratching may spread the ulcers to nearby body areas.
Treatment: Antibiotic drugs.
Special precautions: No intercourse until treatment has been completed and the patient is cured, to prevent spread of the infection.

Charley horse. *See* Muscle cramp.

Chem screen. *See* Sequential multiple analysis.

Chemical burns. *See* Appendix F: First Aid, Burns.

Chemotherapy. The use of one or more chemical agents to treat cancer and certain other diseases. The chemotherapeutic agents are very strong and highly toxic drugs. Some are used locally, on the skin, for example; others may be taken by mouth, or given by injection.

The drugs act by killing cells harmful to the body, such as cancer cells. Unfortunately, many of these agents also kill normal cells. Doctors use various methods to control damage to normal cells, such as planning rest periods between treatments, and using other drugs to protect normal cells. Although chemotherapeutic drugs can be very dangerous, they save the lives of many patients. *See also* Cancer.

Chicken pox (varicella). A highly contagious childhood disease. Adults may become infected if they did not have chicken pox in childhood.
Cause: A type of herpes virus called *Varicella zoster.*
Symptoms: Itchy red rash that turns into small blisters over most of the body. The blisters form crusts that drop off within two weeks.
Treatment: Most patients recover without treatment. An antiviral drug, Zovirax, may shorten the illness if it is used in the early stages of the infection. Anti-itch medications applied locally control discomfort. A chicken-pox vaccine, Varivax, is now available. Children from twelve months to twelve years receive one injection. Teens thirteen and older, as well as adults who have never had chickenpox, receive the vaccine in two injections, four to eight weeks apart.
Special precautions: Because chicken pox is highly contagious, a person who has not had the disease should avoid contact

with an infected child or adult. The disease is no longer contagious once the lesions crust over.

Child abuse. *See* Abuse.

Chiropractic. A practitioner of chiropractic theory uses massage and manipulation of the spine and other parts of the body, with the intent to preserve or restore healthy functioning of the nervous system. No drugs or surgery are used.

Chlamydial infection. A sexually transmitted disease.

Cause: The organism *Chlamydia trachomatis.* Chlamydial infection is today the most common sexually transmitted bacterial disease in American teens ages fifteen to nineteen. There are often no immediate symptoms, but infection can lead to serious complications. The infection can be detected only through laboratory tests. Many infected people are unaware of this infection, and may pass it on to sexual partners. Pregnant women may transmit the infection to their babies.

Transmission: Occurs during sexual intercourse with an infected partner. During pregnancy it is passed on to the unborn baby.

Symptoms in women: None may be apparent, but the infection can be spread to sexual partners. Noticeable symptoms usually include burning on urination and a puslike discharge from the vagina. The cervix may appear red and swollen (visible in an internal examination).

Symptoms in men: None may be apparent, but the infection can be spread to sexual partners. Noticeable symptoms include a watery or mucous discharge from the penis and itching or burning of the urinary tube (urethra), especially while passing urine.

Symptoms in newborn babies: Infection of the membranes covering the eye (conjunctivitis), or pneumonia shortly after birth.

Complications in women:
• Further infections in the genital area
• Acute and chronic pelvic inflammatory disease, with possible damage to reproductive organs
• Possible sterility (inability to have children)
• Arthritis

Complications in men:
• Painful inflammation (epididymitis) of the tube (epididymis) that stores sperm produced by the testicles
• Pain and swelling of the scrotum (the sac that contains the testicles)
• Achy feeling or pain in the lower abdomen or inguinal area (where the thigh joins the abdomen)
• Arthritis

Treatment: Antibiotic drugs and other treatments, depending on symptoms and complications. Hospitalization may be necessary for acutely ill persons.

Special precautions: No sex until treatment is completed.

Cholesterol. A substance present in the blood. Large amounts of cholesterol can form plaques that cause a blockage of major blood vessels, high blood pressure, and heart disease.

Cholesterol profile. A blood test to determine the amount of total cholesterol and several of its fractions. A high blood cholesterol level may contribute to hardening of the arteries and heart disease. High levels of the fraction HDL (high density lipoprotein) protect against heart disease by aiding in the removal of fatty deposits from blood vessel walls. High levels of the fractions LDL (low density lipoprotein) and triglycerides have been associated with heart disease.

Chondromalacia. Weakening of a cartilage. *See* Chondromalacia patella.

Chondromalacia patella. Softening of the knee-cap (patella), with soreness of the thigh muscles and tendons.

Chromosome. The portion of each living cell that contains genes, the tiny units that carry characteristics inherited from one's parents, such as the color of the eyes or hair. Each human being has 46 chromosomes, existing in 23 pairs. The sex chromosomes that pair at the time the mother's egg is fertilized by the father's sperm determine the baby's sex.

Chronic. Lasting a long time; may refer to an illness or other condition that lasts for some period of time. Opposite of Acute.

Chronic fatigue syndrome (CFS). A poorly understood condition that occurs mainly in women ages twenty to forty. Symptoms include constant tiredness, sometimes swollen glands, or mild elevation of body temperature. No specific cause has been found. Treatment is mainly supportive, based on symptoms. It includes rest and a nourishing diet.

Circle jerking. Masturbation among a group of boys or men.

Circulation (blood). The blood's passage, beginning in the left side of the heart, flowing through arteries throughout the body, and returning by way of veins from the body's tissues to the right side of the heart and the lungs, where it is reoxygenated, to resume passage through the body.

The average adult has three to six quarts of blood in his or her body; the heart pumps about 1,250 gallons of blood through the body each day. *See also* Blood; Heart.

Circumcision. Surgical removal of the fore-

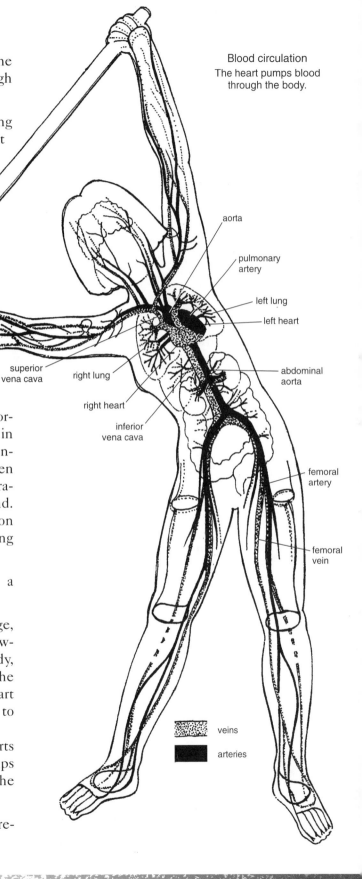

Blood circulation
The heart pumps blood through the body.

aorta

pulmonary artery

left lung

left heart

superior vena cava

right lung

right heart

inferior vena cava

abdominal aorta

femoral artery

femoral vein

veins

arteries

skin of the penis, for cosmetic, health, or religious reasons.

Climax, sexual. *See* Orgasm.

Clitoris. A part of the female genitalia, located above the urinary tube (urethra). The clitoris, similar to the penis, contains erectile tissue that becomes rigid during sexual excitement.

Cocaine. A habit-forming (addictive) chemical substance that makes the user feel high. This feeling does not last long.

People addicted to cocaine often have such a craving for it that they lose all interest in school, job, family, and friends. Because the drug is expensive, users will often steal, rob, or perform other illegal acts to get money so they can stay high.

The dangers of cocaine use include severe mental and physical damage:

Mental damage: Cocaine addicts think they have normal judgment, but in fact, their judgment is very poor. Cocaine users and addicts may become excited, dizzy, and incoherent. They sometimes hear voices and feel depressed, and may become paranoid. They may make bad decisions while driving and in other situations where good judgment is critical.

Physical damage: Cocaine users often have nosebleeds, and permanent damage can occur in the interior structures of the nose when cocaine is snorted over a period of time. A user's veins can be damaged or destroyed by injecting the drug. HIV, hepatitis, and other infections are spread when users share needles to inject cocaine.

Prolonged use of cocaine causes nausea and dizziness, tingling in the hands and feet, a fast pulse, rapid breathing, and dilated pupils. After taking large doses of cocaine a user may develop seizures, an irregular pulse, and heart or breathing problems. In young people, it is also associated with heart attacks. Cocaine use can also cause death. *See also* Crack.

Coitus. Heterosexual intercourse. *See* Sex, heterosexual.

Cold sores. Usually caused by herpes simplex, a type of herpes virus. A cold sore may appear on the lips, or elsewhere on or in the mouth, as one or more fluid-filled blisters that crust after some time and fall off.

Cold sores may occur during a fever, with stress, after exposure to the sun, due to a food allergy, occasionally during menstruation, or after dental treatment. Once a person has had cold sores, they may recur at intervals, usually following one of the situations mentioned above.

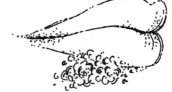

Cold sores first appear as tiny blisters, usually on or near the lips.

Colitis, ulcerative. Chronic inflammation of the large bowel, of unknown cause. Symptoms include cramps, bloody diarrhea, weight loss, and anemia.

Treatment consists of bland meals, replacement of lost blood, and medication to soothe the inflamed bowel wall. Surgery is often the treatment of choice because, depending on age and severity of the condition, it can cure this disease. Surgery may also be recommended because the disease is sometimes associated with eventual colon cancer.

Colon. *See* Intestine.

Color blindness. *See* Eye disorders.

Colostomy. *See* Ostomy.

Colposcopy. A procedure used in diagnosing abnormalities of the cervix. The cervix is painted with acetic acid solution to highlight any unusual lesion, and a colposcope (an instrument fitted with a high-power magnifying glass) is inserted into the vagina to identify problem areas. Any tissue from abnormal-appearing areas is then removed for diagnosis and determination of treatment.

Comedone. A clogged pore in the skin; a blackhead. *See* Acne.

Complete blood count (CBC). A test that measures the number of blood cells (red cells, white cells, and platelets) present in the blood. A low red cell level indicates anemia, a shortage of red blood cells. A low or a high white cell level may point to an infection. A low platelet count may indicate a bleeding problem.

Compulsion, obsessive-compulsive disorder. A person's unreasonable belief, usually based on various irrational fears, that he or she has to behave in a particular way. For example, a person may fear germs so much that he or she becomes obsessed with their danger, washing the hands again and again to get rid of the germs. Other fears may force such people to check dozens of times during the night whether they have locked their doors, or to walk only on one side of the street, because they are afraid to cross to the other side.

Computed tomography, Computerized axial tomography (CAT scan, CT, CTT). *See* CT scan.

Conception. The process during which a man's sperm and a woman's egg (ovum) unite to form a fertilized egg (zygote), the first stage in a pregnancy. A recent study suggests conception is most likely to occur following intercourse during the five days before the woman ovulates, and on the day of ovulation. *See also* Fertilization.

Condom, female. A new contraceptive de-

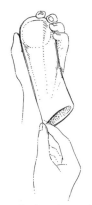
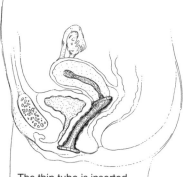

the female condom

The thin tube is inserted into the vagina; the outer rim remains outside.

vice for women. The female condom consists of a plastic pouch that the woman inserts to cover the vagina and cervix, protecting against pregnancy as well as sexually transmitted diseases. *See also* Contraceptive.

Condom, male. A contraceptive device worn over the penis during intercourse to protect against pregnancy, sexually transmitted diseases, and HIV infection. *See also* Contraceptive.

Condoms are made of animal (lamb) skin, rubber, or a rubberlike synthetic substance called latex. Latex is the safest material because it prevents passage of many harmful organisms and other material that may be present in sperm or vaginal fluid. A newly developed product made of polyurethane (Avanti condom) may soon be widely available. It is thinner than a latex condom, less likely to be damaged by certain lubricants, and useful for persons allergic to latex.

Condoms are available in different styles and sizes in drugstores and family planning centers. Here are some guidelines for the use of condoms.

Don't
- Store condoms in a hot place—in the sun or on a radiator, for example—where they may be damaged

How to put on a condom

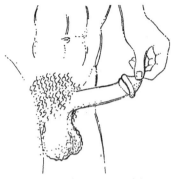

Place condom over the tip of the erect penis.

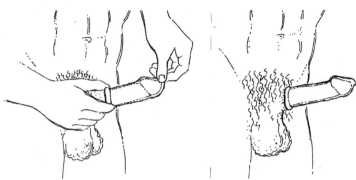

Unroll the condom to the base of the penis. Leave some space at the tip to catch the semen.

The condom in place on the erect penis

- Use old condoms; they may break or tear
- Use an oil-based lubricant such as Vaseline; it destroys condom materials

Do
- Put the condom on well before foreplay or intercourse
- Remove the condom after intercourse, before the penis becomes flaccid (limp)
- Buy only high-quality latex condoms, and follow the package instructions
- Select condoms with a lubricant containing nonoxynol-9, a spermicidal agent

Condylomata acuminata. *See* Genital warts.

Confidential. Kept private, not revealed to others. The results of a confidential laboratory test, for example, are given to the patient only, to ensure privacy.

Congenital. Used to describe a condition, defect, or disease that exists from birth. Congenital conditions may be physical or mental and may develop before or during birth.

Conjunctivitis. Inflammation of the membranes that cover the eye. Caused by irritation, allergy, or infection. Treatment depends on the cause.

Contact dermatitis (allergic dermatitis). A skin reaction, such as a rash, caused by contact with a substance that is irritating or poisonous, or to which the skin is allergic. Treatment includes avoidance of the substance and medications such as a cortisone cream. *See also* Dermatitis; Seborrheic dermatitis.

Contact lens. A thin artificial lens prescribed to correct vision problems such as nearsightedness. The lens fits directly over the eyeball.

Contact lens wearers need to insert the lenses according to instructions. Users must keep the lenses clean, to avoid eye irritations and infections. *See also* Eye disorders.

Contraception. A method used to prevent pregnancy. *See* Contraceptive.

Contraceptive. A device, method, or medication used by a woman or a man to prevent conception and pregnancy.

Barrier contraceptives prevent sperm from reaching an egg and entering it. Therefore the egg cannot be fertilized. Barrier contraceptives include the cervical cap, condom, diaphragm, and the Sponge, which may no longer be available. Each of these is discussed in separate alphabetical entries.

Hormonal contraceptive medications include pills, surgical implants, and injections. These medications consist of hormones that prevent pregnancy in one of three ways: (1)

by preventing the release of an egg from the ovary so that there can be no pregnancy; (2) by acting to form thick mucus at the entrance of the womb (uterus) so that the sperm will not be able to get through; or (3) by thinning out the lining of the womb so that it is too thin to support and nourish a fertilized egg.

Hormonal contraceptives include:

The Pill (oral contraceptive): Widely used by teenage girls and adult women, the oral contraceptive is available only by prescription after a physical examination. The exam ensures that a teen can safely use hormonal pills for a period of time. Anyone taking the pill should have regular checkups as suggested by the physician. *See also* Birth control pill; Oral contraceptive.

Contraceptive implants: In the Norplant System, several (usually six) small capsules filled with contraceptive hormones are surgically inserted under the skin of the upper arm. Implants release a low, continuous dose of hormones to protect against pregnancy for three to five years.

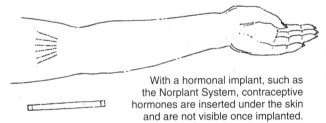

With a hormonal implant, such as the Norplant System, contraceptive hormones are inserted under the skin and are not visible once implanted.

Contraceptive injections: Injections of hormones such as Depo-Provera provide protection against pregnancy for three months at a time.

Contraceptive foam and jelly: These substances contain chemicals with contraceptive properties. They are available in drugstores without prescription. They are most effective when used together with a condom or diaphragm. *See also* Spermicide.

Effectiveness of contraceptive methods

Most effective

- Hormonal implants or long-acting injections
- Oral contraceptives (pill) IUDs
- Condom with spermicide
- Diaphragm with spermicide
- Condom without spermicide
- Diaphragm without spermicide
- Contraceptive sponge
- Cervical cap
- Withdrawal
- Natural (rhythm) method
- Spermicide alone

Least effective

Contraceptive medications for men: Several devices and medications for men are currently under study; none are available for general use.

Convulsion. *See* Seizure.

Corneal abrasion. A scratch or similar injury of the transparent covering (membrane) over the eye.

CPR. *See* Cardiopulmonary resuscitation.

Crabs. *See* Lice, pubic.

Crack. A more dangerous, potent, faster-acting, and cheaper form of cocaine. Crack consists of small crystals ("rocks") that are smoked in a pipe or in a large marijuana cigarette ("blunt"). *See also* Cocaine.

Cramps, menstrual (dysmenorrhea). Abdominal discomfort during a menstrual period. Menstrual discomfort is common. The cramps are caused by chemicals (prostaglandins) in the lining of the uterus that stimulate the uterine muscles to contract. Cramps usually occur only during the first three days of the period. If discomfort lasts longer, consult a health care professional.

What to do if you have cramps:
- Get lots of rest
- Take a warm (not hot) bath

- Use a warm (not hot) heating pad
- Gently rub your abdomen while lying down
- Exercise by doing the pelvic tilt: Stand with your feet about a foot apart, knees bent. Then rock your pelvis forward and back ten to fifteen times. You can also do this exercise lying flat on your back, lifting your pelvis two to three inches off the floor. Count to five before lowering your pelvis. Do this six to eight times
- Try mild over-the-counter pain relievers
- If the milder drugs don't help, your doctor may prescribe a stronger medication

Cramps, muscle. *See* Muscle cramps.

Crohn's disease (regional ileitis). Chronic inflammation of the final part of the small intestine (ileum) or other parts of the intestine. The cause is unknown. The inflammation gradually affects all the layers of the intestinal wall. Symptoms include cramps, diarrhea, fever, abdominal pain, and feeling ill. Treatment includes diet, rest, and medications. *See also* Inflammatory bowel disease.

Cross eye. *See* Eye disorders, strabismus.

Cross-match (X-match). Mixing a small amount of donor blood with the recipient's blood to test for compatibility before giving a blood transfusion.

CT scan. A test that uses special X rays, a computer, and a scanner to produce multiple images of a body area such as a bone, the brain, the kidneys, or an abdominal organ. The images are then recorded on a video display terminal for diagnostic study. A dye may be injected into a vein before the CT scan, so that the part to be studied is more easily visible.

Culture. A laboratory procedure done on blood or other body fluids to detect the presence of infection. A sample of blood or other body fluid is placed in a nourishing broth or other substance, where the organisms can grow and multiply. The laboratory technician identifies harmful organisms and reports them to the doctor, who prescribes specific antibiotics to treat the infection.

Cunnilingus. Sexual activity in which the partner's mouth is in contact with the female's genitals.

Cyst. A sac consisting of tissue and filled with fluid. A cyst may appear inside or on the body's surface. Depending on the cyst's origin and location, the fluid may be blood, sweat, lymph, or a glandular secretion. The cyst may disappear without treatment or may require removal by a doctor. *See also* Sebaceous cyst.

Cystic fibrosis (CF). A chronic, inherited disease. This disease affects the sweat- and mucus-producing glands. Poor functioning of these glands in turn causes abnormal functioning of the lungs, the digestive system, and the reproductive system.

Cystoscopy. A test to determine the presence of a problem or abnormality in the urinary tube (urethra) or in the bladder.

Cytomegalovirus (CMV). A virus that causes infection in various parts of the body. Infection may occur at any age, with or without symptoms, even in newborn infants who are infected by their mothers. Sometimes the infection is caused by a transfusion of blood that contains the virus. The person receiving the transfusion may develop a fever that lasts for several weeks, inflammation of the liver, and other symptoms.

CMV infection may lead to pneumonia, with symptoms (cough, fever) appearing gradually over several days. Diagnosis is made by examining body fluids. There is no specific treatment. CMV infection is sometimes confused with mononucleosis, another viral infection. *See also* Mononucleosis.

D

Dandruff. *See* Seborrheic dermatitis.

Date rape. Sexual intercourse forced on a date. In date rape, a partner misinterprets or ignores the other partner's wishes. Use of alcohol or other substances that affect judgment and self-control may play a part in date rape. Whatever the cause, date rape is always a crime, and a person who commits date rape should be reported to the authorities.

Deafness (hearing loss). Partial or total inability to hear with one or both ears. Deafness has many causes: the ears may be filled with wax, which can be removed by an ear irrigation; or they may be filled with water, after swimming. Shaking the head first to one side, then to the other, allows water to drain from each ear.

More serious causes of hearing loss include infection acquired during fetal life or shortly after birth: for example, infection of the mother during pregnancy with German measles; a congenital nervous system defect; side effects of certain medications; trauma such as punctured eardrums, or other injury to the ear and surrounding structures that occur during an accident.

A person with impaired hearing needs to be examined by an ear, nose, and throat (ENT) specialist, who determines the cause, as well as the extent of hearing loss with an audiogram. Treatment depends on the cause, and includes medication, a hearing aid, or surgery.

Dehydration. Inadequate water content in the body's tissues. A person may become dehydrated due to: sweating while exercising; an illness, especially if it involves a fever; diarrhea or vomiting; excessive urination due to diabetes; inability or lack of desire to drink enough fluids; or exposure to hot temperatures.

Any of these conditions may cause excessive loss of water from body tissues, and lead to serious results. For example, an infant who becomes dehydrated as a result of diarrhea may die, unless treated promptly with fluids (usually given intravenously).

Dehydration can be prevented by drinking six to eight glasses of water and other fluids a day under ordinary circumstances; more is needed if circumstances cause a greater loss of water. If dehydration is caused by disease, the disease must be treated.

Delirium. A state of severe confusion caused by such conditions as a high fever; severe inflammation of the brain; abuse of toxic substances that affect the brain, such as alcohol, barbiturates, and other drugs of abuse, especially when a person suddenly decides to stop (withdraw from) drinking alcohol or using drugs; and certain diseases that involve deterioration of the brain.

Symptoms of delirium include severe confusion; irritability; agitation; inability to recognize the time, place, or familiar events normally readily identified; hallucinations (erroneous beliefs that certain circumstances, situations, shapes, or people exist that in reality are not there, or not in the form perceived).

Treatment depends on the cause. Medications such as sedatives and other drugs may be given to control the mental effects. Other medications are prescribed to reduce a high fever. Oral or intravenous fluids may be given to persons dehydrated by a high fever.

Patients who are in delirium must be carefully observed, to protect them from hurting themselves or others. Restraints may be needed.

Dementia. A mental disorder marked by a

loss of memory and inability to function normally. Dementia may be caused by an infection of the brain such as encephalitis or meningitis, a tumor, or certain drugs and chemicals, or it may be a result of aging. The disorder may be a sign of a psychological disturbance such as schizophrenia. In older people, dementia may be a sign of Alzheimer's disease.

Dental braces. *See* Braces, dental.

Dental care. Good dental care includes brushing the teeth at least twice daily, flossing the teeth every day, and having a checkup and cleaning by a dentist twice a year. *See also* Teeth.

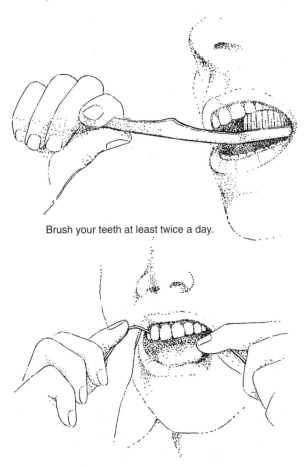

Brush your teeth at least twice a day.

Use dental floss daily to remove food particles between your teeth.

Dental caries. Cavities, or areas of decay, in the teeth. Caries often develop when dental hygiene is neglected. *See* Dental care.

Dental flossing. Cleaning between the teeth with a length of thick waxed or unwaxed thread.

Dental rubber dam. A thin piece of a rubberlike substance called latex, used by dentists to isolate the specific tooth they are working on. May be used to prevent transmission of infections during cunnilingus.

Deoxyribonucleic acid. *See* DNA.

Depo-Provera. A long-acting contraceptive drug that contains the hormone progesterone. When injected intramuscularly by a health professional, Depo-Provera prevents pregnancy for three months. The drug works by preventing ovulation (release of an egg). It is highly effective (99 percent), and especially helpful for women with chronic health problems such as diabetes or epilepsy. The injection must be repeated after three months to provide continuous pregnancy prevention. *See also* Contraceptive.

Depression. A disturbance of thought, mood, or behavior. Depression is a common problem among young people. Symptoms include:
- Feelings of worthlessness
- Lack of hope for the future
- Lack of energy
- Loss of interest in activities
- Inability to find pleasure
- Overeating or undereating
- Oversleeping or insomnia

People who suffer from depression in its severest forms may want or attempt to kill themselves. A depression may be triggered by these factors:
- Genetic causes
- A disturbance of nerve transmitters in the brain

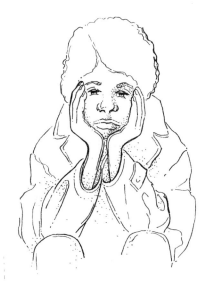
Sadness, sleep disorders, hopelessness, and fatigue may be signs of depression.

- A significant loss such as the death of a parent or close friend, or the breakup of a relationship

Some young people turn to drugs, alcohol, or sex in an attempt to feel less distraught, but these measures rarely help for long. Young people who are depressed should promptly seek counseling and treatment.

Dermabrasion. Scraping of the top layers of skin; a technique used by a dermatologist, a specialist in skin diseases, to smooth away skin scarred by acne.

Dermatitis. Inflammation of the skin. There are various types of dermatitis and many different causes. *See also* Contact dermatitis; Seborrheic dermatitis.

Deviated septum. The septum, the bone that divides the nose vertically into halves, is normally straight or nearly straight. An injury may fracture or damage the septum. When the injury heals, the nose may have a crooked, or deviated, shape that may cause breathing difficulties. Surgery can correct the problem. *See also* Rhinoplasty.

Diabetes insipidus. A hormonal disorder that affects the pituitary gland in the brain. The most common cause is trauma. Symptoms include passing very large amounts of urine, up to twenty quarts or more each twenty-four hours. The fluid loss, in turn, leads to great thirst and, often, dehydration. Treatment consists of fluid replacement, administration of antidiuretic hormone, either through nose drops or injection, and treatment of the underlying condition.

Diabetes mellitus. An endocrine disorder in which the body is either unable to produce sufficient insulin, or is unable to utilize the insulin it produces. Insulin helps the body utilize sugar (glucose) and fats (lipids). In people with diabetes, the muscles and other body tissues cannot use sugar and fats effectively. Excess sugar and fats build up in the blood and in other parts of the body, creating many health problems. *See also* Insulin.

Symptoms of diabetes include excessive thirst, hunger, and urination; weight loss; mental confusion; and many other complications.

There are two main types of diabetes mellitus. Type 1 diabetes (juvenile onset or insulin dependent) occurs mainly in children and adolescents (IDDM: Insulin dependent diabetes mellitus type 1). This form requires regular administration of insulin for survival. Type 2 diabetes (adult onset or non-insulin dependent) occurs in adults, often associated with obesity (NIDDM: non-insulin dependent diabetes mellitus type 2). This form may or may not require insulin. In many patients it may be controlled by diet, oral medication, exercise, or a combination of these.

Diagnosis. The process of determining a specific condition or disease. *See also* Symptoms.

Diaphragm, anatomic. A muscle located between the lungs and the abdomen that helps the lungs to expand and contract.

How to insert a diaphragm

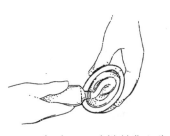

Apply spermicidal jelly to the rim and interior of the diaphragm.

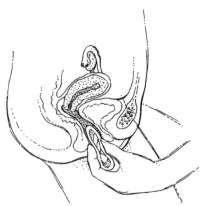

Compress the diaphragm to insert it into the vagina.

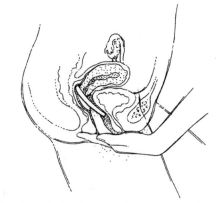

Gently push the diaphragm into place, covering the cervix.

Diaphragm, contraceptive. A dome-shaped device made of latex. It is inserted in the vagina and placed over the cervix, the entrance to the womb. Used correctly, a properly fitting diaphragm blocks sperm and so prevents pregnancy.

A diaphragm is prescribed and fitted by a health professional. A spermicidal (sperm-killing) jelly, placed in the diaphragm before insertion, further aids in preventing pregnancy. *See also* Contraceptive.

Diarrhea. Frequent, very soft or liquid bowel movements. The usual cause is a viral or bacterial infection in the intestine; other causes may be an allergy or a reaction to a drug, or it may result from eating certain foods, for example, an excess of fruit. Mild diarrhea is treated with a soft diet, and an over-the-counter antidiarrheal drug such as Imodium or Pepto-Bismol, if needed. Do not use these medications if there is blood in the stool. Severe diarrhea lasting more than a few days requires a medical checkup and diagnostic tests to find the cause. Treatment consists of antibiotics or other drugs to fight a diagnosed infection; oral or intravenous fluids containing electrolytes (substances that maintain the body's acid/base balance) to re-place fluid lost by diarrhea and restore normal cell function throughout the body, and bed rest. If severe, hospitalization may be needed.

Diet. The food and liquids a person consumes each day. A nutritious daily diet includes selections from the five major food groups. *See* Food groups.

> **For a healthy diet**
> - Include a variety of foods
> - Maintain a healthy weight
> - Follow a low-fat diet
> - Eat plenty of vegetables, fruits, and whole-grain products
> - Use salt and sugar moderately
> - Limit your consumption of alcohol

Digestion. The breakdown of food on its way through the digestive tract (mouth, esophagus, stomach, and intestines), to allow the absorption of nutrients and elimination of waste.

Digestive system. The group of organs and tissues that process foods for use by the body. It includes the digestive tract (a long tube that extends from the mouth to the rectum), the liver, and the pancreas.

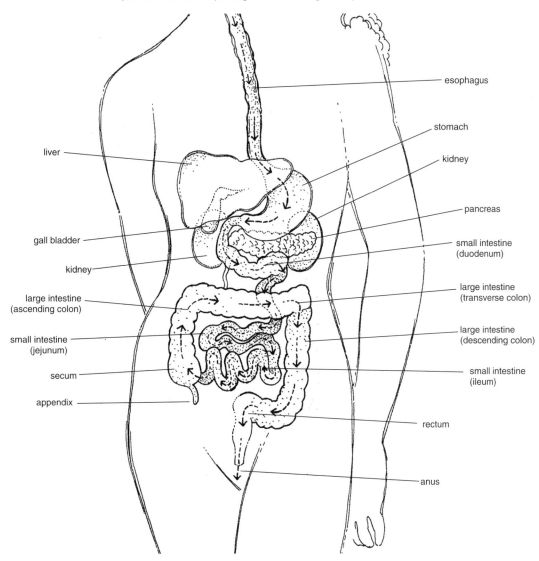

the digestive system
(arrows indicate the passage of food through the system)

esophagus

stomach

kidney

pancreas

small intestine
(duodenum)

large intestine
(transverse colon)

large intestine
(descending colon)

small intestine
(ileum)

rectum

anus

liver

gall bladder

kidney

large intestine
(ascending colon)

small intestine
(jejunum)

secum

appendix

Dilation and curettage (D&C). A procedure carried out by a physician to remove the contents of the uterus during an abortion or following a miscarriage. The procedure is also used to identify abnormalities of the uterus. *See also* Abortion.

Dilation and evacuation. *See* Abortion.

Diphtheria. A very dangerous bacterial throat infection caused by the organism *Corynebacterium diphtheriae*. It occurs in children who have not been vaccinated against this disease. Adults who have not been vaccinated and who never had diphtheria in childhood may contract the disease from an infected child or adult.

Diphtheria can cause a blockage in the back of the throat, making breathing difficult or impossible. Death may result if the blockage is not relieved. Diphtheria vaccine given during infancy will protect a person for life. *See also* Immunization.

Diplopia. *See* Eye disorders, Double vision.

Discharge. Fluid produced somewhere in the body and emerging from a body opening. The color, odor, and amount are significant. A discharge may be normal, or it may indicate an infection, especially if it comes from the vagina, the penis, or the eyes.

Dislocation (bone). Change of a bone's normal position after it has slipped out of its joint. A dislocation is generally the result of trauma such as a sports injury or an accident.

DNA. A constituent in the nucleus of every living cell. DNA contains the genetic material that allows reproduction of other cells of the same kind.

Double vision. *See* Eye disorders.

Douche. A method of cleansing the vagina with a solution. Douches are not effective contraceptives. Douches can be made at home with vinegar and water, or they may be prepared solutions containing various chemicals and fragrances.

The liquid is placed in a small douche bag attached to a tube ending in a nozzle. The nozzle is inserted into the vagina, and the liquid flows through the tube and nozzle, to irrigate the vaginal area. Douching is rarely necessary because the body has its own natural cleansing methods. In fact, it can upset the balance of organisms that normally live in the vagina, and harmful yeast organisms may multiply and start an infection.

A woman who develops a vaginal discharge should see a doctor to find out if an infection is present. She should not use a douche before the examination, as the doctor may not then be able to see the discharge and find its cause.

Down syndrome. An inherited condition caused by an extra chromosome. A child with Down syndrome suffers from mental retardation that ranges from mild to severe. Indications of the condition include slanted eyes, an unusually long crease in the palms of the hands, a flattened bridge of the nose, muscular weakness, and sometimes heart disease.

Downer. *See* Tranquilizer.

Drug abuse. The unnecessary or excessive use of a substance such as cigarettes, alcohol, cocaine, heroin, or marijuana, which may lead to physical or psychological dependence on that substance. Drug abuse may cause serious physical and mental symptoms.

A person who can't get through the day without using one or more of these substances is an addict. Addicts may spend most of the day planning how to get enough of the substance to satisfy the constant craving for it. An addict may become physically ill without the substance amount needed to get high.

Treatment and recovery from severe substance abuse is a long, complicated process. It is not successful unless the addict sincerely wants to change. *See* Appendix A: Hotlines.

Drug overdose. Taking an excessive amount of an over-the-counter or prescription medication. *See* Appendix B.

Dwarfism. A condition that results in extremely short stature. Dwarfism may be caused by an inability of the bones and cartilage to form properly. In some cases, dwarfism is an inherited problem.

Dyslexia. A term that refers to reading disorders. While people with dyslexia are often average or above average in intelligence, they have difficulty learning reading, writing, and other skills. With special teaching techniques, many individuals can be helped to master the tasks. *See also* Learning disabled.

Dysmenorrhea. *See* Cramps, menstrual.

Dyspnea. Difficulty in breathing. This may occur as a result of being at a high altitude (where the air is thinner and contains less oxygen), a lung problem, certain types of heart disease, and various other conditions, such as anxiety or poor physical stamina.

A healthy person who has difficulty breathing at high altitudes usually adjusts within a few hours. During that time, it is wise to avoid exertion until the body becomes used to the different atmospheric conditions. Difficulty in breathing caused by an illness must be treated by managing the underlying illness.

Dysuria. A burning sensation while urinating; often occurs during an infection of the urinary or genitourinary tract.

Ear irrigation. A treatment to remove wax plugging the ear canal. *See* Ear wax.

Ear piercing. *See* Piercing, body.

Ear wax (cerumen). The waxy substance present in the ears. Most people normally have a small amount of wax in one or both ears, which does not interfere with hearing or require removal. Some people accumulate larger amounts of wax in their ears, which interferes with good hearing. A doctor can perform a painless procedure called an ear irrigation to remove the excess wax. Commercially available products such as Debrox or hydrogen peroxide are also used to reduce wax build-up in the ears.

Warning signs of an eating disorder
- Restricting calorie intake severely, perhaps to 500 calories a day
- Skipping two or more meals a day, or eating only on alternate days
- Eating very large amounts of food in a short period, while feeling out of control
- Eating large amounts of food when not hungry
- Using laxatives, diuretics, forced vomiting, or other purging behaviors to control weight
- Overexercising to control weight
- Avoiding social situations that involve food
- Limiting social activities to maintain an eating or exercise schedule
- A preoccupation with food and weight
- A feeling of self-disgust, guilt, or depression after overeating

---

Eating disorders. Anorexia nervosa, bulimia, and binge eating, grouped as eating disorders, are among the most common serious illnesses of teenagers and young adults. They generally appear during adolescence and, unless successfully treated, may have serious medical and psychological consequences. *See also* Anorexia nervosa; Binge; Bulimia.

Echocardiogram. An ultrasound test to determine the presence of abnormal structures and dysfunctions of the heart.

Ectopic pregnancy. *See* Tubal pregnancy.

Eczema. A chronic, inflammatory skin condition. Eczema may redden the skin or produce scales, pustules, crusts, or scabs. A watery discharge, itching, or burning may also be present. The cause of eczema is unknown. People with dry or very thin skin may be more likely to develop eczema.

Ejaculate. *See* Semen.

Ejaculation. The discharge of semen from the penis during sexual climax (orgasm).

Electric shock. *See* Appendix F: First Aid.

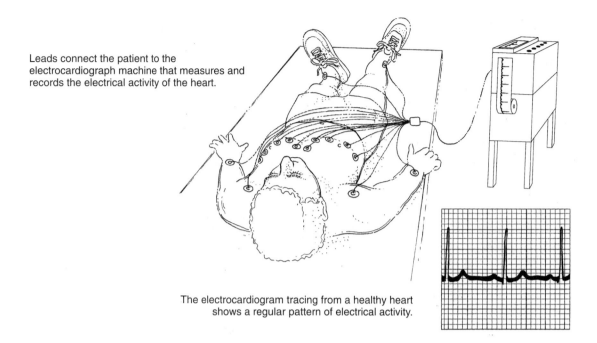

Leads connect the patient to the electrocardiograph machine that measures and records the electrical activity of the heart.

The electrocardiogram tracing from a healthy heart shows a regular pattern of electrical activity.

Electrocardiogram (ECG, EKG). A test to examine the electrical activity of the heart. Wires are placed on the chest, arms, and legs. The heart's electrical patterns are traced and recorded by a machine called an electrocardiograph. The patterns are then examined for abnormal heart rhythms. If any are found, the problem can be identified and treated.

Electroencephalogram (EEG). A test to diagnose electrical activity of the brain. Wires are placed in various positions on the head. Brain waves are traced and recorded by a machine called an encephalograph. The brain wave patterns indicate if brain function is normal. These patterns aid in the diagnosis of brain disease.

Electromyogram (EMG). A test to evaluate muscle function. Electrodes are placed in certain muscles of the arms or legs. Muscle function is observed as the muscles contract and relax; electrical stimulation of the muscles allows study of any abnormalities in nerve conduction.

Electroshock therapy (EST). A treatment for people with depression who have not been helped by medication or other treatment. EST is performed by passing an electric current through the brain while the patient is sedated or anesthesized. After the treatment, some patients may be drowsy, and have a poor memory for recent events. This is generally temporary. A series of EST treatments are given to achieve satisfactory results.

ELISA (Enzyme-linked immunosorbent assay). A blood test to find and measure substances such as hormones, drugs, or HIV antibodies; such antibodies would indicate HIV infection.

Embryo. The developing baby during the first three months of pregnancy. After that time the baby is called a fetus. *See also* Pregnancy.

Emesis. *See* Vomiting.

Emphysema. A chronic illness that damages and destroys lung tissues. Emphysema often occurs in adults who have smoked for many years. Long-term smoking can cause irreversible lung damage, with frequent coughing and difficulty in breathing.

A person with advanced emphysema has so little breath (oxygen) available that even mild exertion such as walking or climbing a flight of stairs is difficult or impossible. There is no cure for this disease. Medication is used to keep remaining lung tissues clear of mucus. Use of a portable oxygen supply allows performance of essential daily activities.

Encephalitis. An inflammation of brain cells, most often caused by a virus. Encephalitis may develop as a complication of a childhood infectious disease such as measles or mumps; other cases of encephalitis may follow mononucleosis or herpes simplex infection. HIV infection may lead to the development of encephalitis, as, occasionally, may Lyme disease.

Symptoms depend on the severity of the infection, and may include general feelings of illness, fever, headache, weakness, and a loss of appetite. If the infection is more severe, the patient may show irritability and restlessness, speech impairment, loss of muscle function, and drowsiness progressing to coma in a very severe case.

A diagnosis is made by means of a CAT scan or MRI, analysis of spinal fluid, and various blood tests. Drugs are then given that fight the specific organisms that cause the disease. Some viruses do not respond to any currently known drugs. Patients in this situation are treated with supportive measures. Recovery may be slow and, as with other brain injuries, the patient may require rehabilitative treatment over a period of time.

Endocrine gland. A gland that produces a hormone and discharges it directly into the bloodstream. Endocrine glands include the pituitary gland (in the brain), the thyroid gland (neck), the pancreas and adrenal glands (abdomen), the testes, and the ovaries (lower abdominal region). *See also* Gland.

Endodontia. A branch of dentistry that specializes in problems of dental pulp and nearby tissues, such as root canals.

Endometriosis. A disease in which cells normally found in the lining of a woman's uterus (womb) travel to various other parts of her body. The traveling cells may move farther into the muscular layers of the uterus or into the fallopian tubes and the ovaries. Endometriosis cells may migrate to the urinary bladder, intestines, and occasionally even to the lungs. When these cells settle in a place where they don't belong, they interfere with normal function in that organ or body part.

Endometriosis in the reproductive tract (uterus, fallopian tubes, or ovaries) may affect the pain cycle (cramps) of a woman's period. Cramps may start before her period, get worse while it lasts, and continue even after the menstrual (blood) flow stops. The cause of endometriosis is not known.

Endometritis. Inflammation of the lining of the womb.

Endometrium. The tissue membrane that lines the womb.

Endoscopy. A procedure in which a tube (endoscope), sometimes fitted with a light or other devices, is inserted through a body opening to detect problems such as bleeding, a growth, or other abnormal conditions in various parts of the body. An endoscopic examination may be done to examine:
- The food tube (esophagus), stomach, and small intestine
- The breathing tube (trachea), to examine the respiratory tract and the lungs
- The rectum, to diagnose a problem there or in the bowel

A piece of tissue may be removed (biopsy) through the endoscope to aid in diagnosis.

Enema. A procedure in which a certain amount of fluid is inserted into a person's rectum, then allowed to run out. The fluid may consist of warm, soapy water, or a prescribed solution, available at drugstores. An enema may be given for constipation, or in preparation for a diagnostic or surgical procedure that requires a clean, empty bowel.

Enuresis (bed-wetting). Urination during sleep. This is normal for infants and small children who are not yet toilet-trained. An older child or teenager may have an occasional accident caused by anxiety or tension, but frequent bed-wetting indicates a problem.

The difficulty may be physical, as in a urinary tract infection; or there may be an abnormality in the urinary tract or in the nervous system. In some cases, bed-wetting is caused by a behavioral disturbance.

Treatment for younger children includes the use of alarms or sensing devices (behavior modification). Older children may be treated with medications. A medical checkup is necessary to find the cause and provide effective treatment.

Enzyme. A substance, made by body tissue, that produces chemical changes in nutrients such as sugar, and converts them into simpler substances the body's tissues can absorb and use for nourishment or energy.

Enzyme-linked immunosorbent assay (ELISA). *See* ELISA.

Epididymis. A tube that is part of the male reproductive system. It is attached to the testicle, where it collects sperm produced there. *See illustration* The Human Body.

Epididymitis. Inflammation of the epididymis; often caused by a sexually transmitted disease such as gonorrhea or chlamydial infection. Epididymitis may be painful. It requires a prompt search for the infectious cause, and antibiotic treatment. Immediate treatment helps in several ways. It prevents:

- Spread of the infection to a healthy sexual partner
- Damage to the genital tract and the urinary tract
- Sterility (inability to have a child)

Epilepsy. A brain disorder that can cause temporary loss of consciousness and convulsions (seizures). Epilepsy can be controlled by drug therapy. *See also* Seizure. For emergency treatment, *see* Appendix F: First Aid, Seizures.

Epstein-Barr virus (EBV). The virus that causes mononucleosis. *See also* Mononucleosis.

Erection. The hardening of the penis during male sexual excitement. Erectile tissues inside the penis fill with blood (become engorged), to allow sexual intercourse. After climax, the extra blood drains from the erectile tissues, and the penis becomes soft (flaccid) again.

Erogenous zone. A body area that causes sexual feelings or arousal when stimulated.

The genital area and the breasts are the main erogenous zones. Rubbing or caressing various other body areas, such as the ears, the back, or the feet may also arouse sexual excitement.

Erythrocyte sedimentation rate (ESR). A test on blood to determine how much time the red blood cells (erythrocytes) in freshly drawn blood need to settle at the bottom of a test tube.

This test is used when inflammation or infection is suspected. The more red blood cells that settle (sedimentation rate) in one hour, the stronger the likelihood that inflammation or infection is present somewhere in the body.

Esophagoscopy. *See* Endoscopy.

Esophagus (food tube). The tube that carries food from the back of the throat down to the stomach. *See also* Digestive system.

Estrogen. A hormone produced mainly by the ovaries and the adrenal glands.

Exchange transfusion. A treatment in which most of a person's blood supply is gradually replaced. During this procedure, some blood is removed and replaced with donor blood. The process is repeated several times until most of the patient's blood has been replaced. Exchange transfusion can save a baby born with a blood disease caused by the mother's Rh-negative blood reaction against the infant's Rh-positive blood. *See also* Rh factor.

Exocrine gland. A gland that produces a hormone and discharges it through tiny tubes to nearby areas. *See also* Glands.

External genitalia. The visible parts of the male or female genitalia. In men these include the penis and the testicles. In women they include the labia majora (the large, outer lips of the vagina), the labia minora (the smaller inner lips of the vagina), and the clitoris (the small hood above the urinary opening). *See illustration* The Human Body.

Eye disorders.

Color blindness. Inability to differentiate between colors. A person with this condition may not be able to tell blue from black, or one shade of red or green from another shade of the same color. This disorder is caused by a lack of light-sensitive materials that is usually inherited, and more common in men than in women. Most forms of color blindness are relatively mild. There is no treatment.

Nearsightedness (myopia). An eye disorder in which objects close by are seen easily, but more distant objects are blurred. This happens because the distance from the front to the back of the eye is too long for an image to focus on the retina; instead, focusing occurs in front of the retina, causing blurred vision. Prescription eyeglasses or contact lenses correct this problem. Keratotomy, a surgical procedure developed in recent years, is performed for some people with nearsightedness.

Farsightedness (hypermetropia). An eye disorder in which objects are focused behind the retina, blurring close-up objects, while

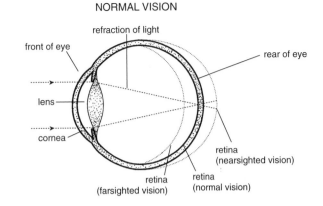

NORMAL VISION

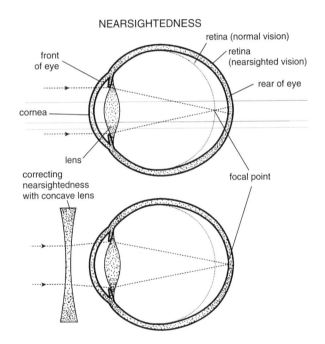

NEARSIGHTEDNESS

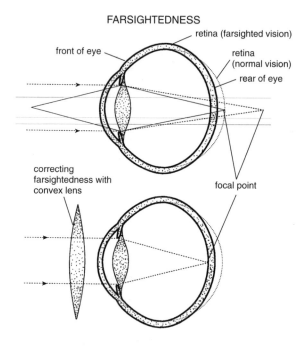

FARSIGHTEDNESS

retina (farsighted vision)

front of eye

retina
(normal vision)

rear of eye

correcting
farsightedness with
convex lens

focal point

ASTIGMATISM

front of eye

Horizontal plane
out of focus

rear of eye

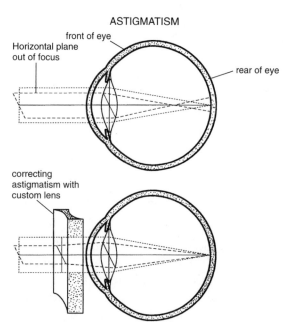

correcting
astigmatism with
custom lens

distant objects can be seen more clearly. A young person with this problem can usually accommodate (ciliary muscles surrounding the pupil dilate or contract it as needed to see an object clearly), but eye strain may de-velop. Prescription eyeglasses or contact lenses correct this problem.

Astigmatism. An eye disorder caused by an irregular curvature of the frontal (cornea) area of the eye, which distorts vision. Prescription eyeglasses or contact lenses compensate for the distortion and correct this problem.

Stye. An infection in the hair follicle of an eyelash. The edge of the eyelid becomes red, swollen, and painful at the site of the infected hair follicle. Yellowish-white pus develops inside, and moves to the top of the swelling. Pain and swelling persist until the stye bursts open and the pus drains out. Treatment includes application of warm (water) compresses, which hastens the rupturing of the stye. If the problem persists or recurs, antibiotic medications are needed.

Double vision (diplopia). A person may see one object doubly as a result of weakness of eye nerves or muscles. Prescription eyeglasses or contact lenses correct this problem.

Strabismus (squint, cross eye, walleye). An eye disorder in which the eyes do not focus on the same object at the same time. Instead, the eyes focus inward (squint), toward the nose (cross-eye), or outward in opposite directions (walleye). This disorder is caused by weak eye muscles. It may be corrected by eye exercises, patching the eye, prescription glasses, contact lenses, and eye medication. Surgery may be needed to correct the problem

Fad diet. A weight loss program that includes only certain kinds of food. Most fad diets are not well balanced and are not healthful if followed for any length of time.

One fad diet, for example, consists only of large quantities of grapefruit. Supposedly this decreases the appetite, and therefore fewer high-calorie foods are required to satisfy hunger. Concentrating exclusively on weight loss at the expense of a well-balanced diet results in poor nutrition. After a time, an inadequate diet will cause major medical problems.

Fallopian tubes. Two slender tubes, each attached to one side of the uterus (womb). *See illustration* The Human Body.

False negative. A negative test result in a person who does have the disease. Inaccurate test results may be due to faulty laboratory methods or an error in writing the report. In fact, no test is 100 percent accurate. Occasionally a false negative result may mean that the test itself is not accurate.

False positive. A positive test result in a person who does not have the disease. Inaccurate test results may be due to inaccurate laboratory methods or an error in writing the report. No test is 100 percent accurate. Occasionally a false positive result may mean that the test itself is not accurate.

Farsightedness. *See* Eye disorders.

Fast food. Foods such as hamburgers or pizza that are quickly prepared and eaten. Fast foods eaten regularly in place of more nourishing meals may provide a poorly balanced diet, since they often contain high levels of sodium, cholesterol, and fats.

Fasting blood sugar (FBS). A blood sample taken from a person who has eaten nothing for at least six to eight hours, to determine the content of sugar in blood.

Fellatio. Oral sexual activity in which a male places his penis inside another person's mouth for sexual gratification.

Female condom. *See* Condom, female.

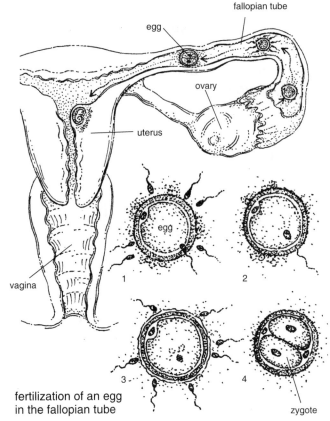

fertilization of an egg
in the fallopian tube

After the egg is released from the ovary into the fallopian tube (top):

1. Many sperm surround the egg
2. One sperm penetrates the outer layer of the egg.
3. The sperm nucleus moves inside the egg. No other sperm can enter.
4. The sperm nucleus and egg nucleus combine and the cell divides into two, now called a zygote.

The zygote travels to the uterus where it implants in the wall to begin a pregnancy.

Fertilization. Penetration of an egg by a sperm, following sexual intercourse or artificial insemination; the first step in starting a pregnancy.

Fetal alcohol syndrome (FAS). A serious illness of newborn babies whose mothers frequently drank substantial amounts of alcohol while pregnant. These babies may be born with many serious, lifelong health problems, including mental retardation, nervous diseases, and heart problems. *See also* Alcohol.

Fetus. The developing unborn baby from the third month of pregnancy until birth.

Fever of unknown origin (FUO). A fever of which the cause has not been determined.

Fibrocystic disease. A condition in which noncancerous lumps appear in a woman's breasts.

First Aid. *See* Appendix F: First Aid.

Flora. Microscopic organisms such as bacteria or viruses that live in the body, or various parts of the body.

Flu (influenza, grippe). A virus infection that causes symptoms such as fever, headache, an achy feeling, sore throat, cough, and a lack of appetite. Mild flu requires rest, fluids, and a pain reliever such as Tylenol for headache. More serious flu cases may require prescribed medication (antibiotics) to prevent a secondary infection, such as a bacterial infection, that can lead to bronchitis or pneumonia, or other complications.

Flu occurs most frequently in the winter and can spread quickly, even causing an epidemic. Depending on the nature of the flu virus, the infection may be mild or severe. People at risk of becoming seriously ill if they develop flu (including teens with asthma, those who smoke heavily, and those who have cancer or a chronic illness such as diabetes) should receive a flu vaccine before the winter begins to allow time to develop immunity against the virus.

Follicle-stimulating hormone (FSH). A hormone produced by the pituitary gland in the brain, which stimulates the production of eggs (ova) in women and sperm in men.

Fondling. Touching or caressing another person's body; may also mean touching the genitals. Fondling is a normal part of foreplay and sex play between partners, provided each partner agrees to these activities. Fondling against a person's wishes is a form of sexual abuse.

Fondling of a child or young teen should be reported to a responsible adult who can stop it and prevent its repetition.

Food and Drug Administration (FDA). The government agency responsible for monitoring the safety and effectiveness of all food and drug products sold in the United States.

Food groups. The five major food categories are (1) grains, (2) vegetables, (3) fruits, (4) dairy products, and (5) meats, dried beans, eggs, and nuts. A well-balanced diet requires the daily intake of a specific number of servings from each category. Guides to a healthy diet are available in health clinics, from your doctor, and in health magazines and books. *See also* Food pyramid.

Food poisoning. Food poisoning is usually caused by eating or drinking food, water, or other liquids contaminated by infectious or-

---

Some common types of food poisoning

Staphylococcus poisoning is caused by eating food contaminated by staphylococcus bacteria. The bacteria have an opportunity to grow when food is prepared and then left standing without refrigeration, as may happen at a picnic. If symptoms are severe, or persist, medical help is needed.

Salmonella poisoning is caused by eating food contaminated with salmonella bacteria. This occurs most often with raw or not fully cooked poultry, fish, meat, and eggs. Mild cases usually clear up by themselves; more severe or long-lasting cases should be seen by a doctor.

Listeria poisoning is caused by bacteria that are found in soil and water, and may cause illness when consumed in large amounts, perhaps from soft blue-veined cheeses or unwashed, raw vegetables. Healthy people usually recover from this type of food poisoning without treatment.

Botulism is a rare but very serious, often fatal, form of food poisoning. It is caused by a Clostridium bacterium that may produce a toxin in improperly canned or preserved food. If the food is fully heated (to 212° F), the toxin is destroyed. Botulism symptoms include blurred vision, and muscle weakness or paralysis, in addition to the other food poisoning symptoms. Botulism requires immediate medical attention.

ganisms such as bacteria. The symptoms—nausea, vomiting, diarrhea, and abdominal pain—can appear almost immediately after eating or drinking the spoiled substance, or up to a day later. *See* Appendix F: First Aid, Food Poisoning.

Food pyramid. An easy guide to healthy eating based on the U.S. Department of Agriculture's "Eating Right Pyramid." The pyramid contains five food groups that should be included in a healthy daily diet: (1) grains, (2) vegetables, (3) fruits, (4) dairy, (5) meats, dried beans, eggs, and nuts. The Food Pyramid illustration shows the types of foods and number of servings of each group to include in the daily diet.

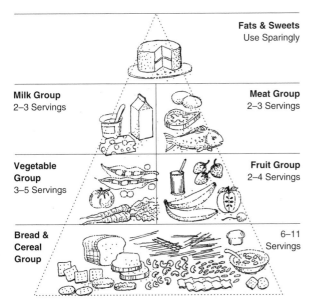

The food pyramid

Foreign body. A substance lodged in some part of the body (eye, ear, rectum, vagina) where it doesn't belong. The foreign body may enter accidentally (a speck of dust in the eye); or as a result of intentional activity (a child pushes a bean or button into an ear, nose, or other body cavity), or as the result of physical assault, where an object is forcibly inserted. A foreign body should be removed by a physician if there is a possibility of tissue damage or other injury.

Foreplay. Various activities performed before sexual intercourse to increase sexual desire. Foreplay may include kissing, fondling, and caressing.

Foreskin. Skin that covers the glans (tip) of the uncircumcised penis. *See also* Circumcision.

Fornication. Sexual intercourse between unmarried people.

Fracture. A break in one or more bones caused by a fall, accident, or illness. *See* Appendix F: First Aid.

Frostbite. *See* Appendix F: First Aid.

Fungal infection. An infection caused by the invasion of a fungus or fungal organism. Common fungal infections of the skin include ringworm, jock itch, and athlete's foot.

In people with a weak or suppressed immune system, fungal organisms may cause serious infections of the mouth or intestinal tract. Fungal infections sometimes involve the respiratory tract or the brain, which may lead to death.

Depending on the location and extent of a fungal infection, both over-the-counter and prescription antifungal medications are used as treatment. *See* Appendix B: Medications

Fungus, fungi (pl). Various forms of mold

that may cause diseases. *See also* Fungal infection.

Furuncle. *See* Abscess.

G

Galactorrhea. Excessive flow of milk from the breast, a normal occurrence during pregnancy and while nursing an infant. At other times, galactorrhea may be a side effect of certain drugs or a symptom of a disorder that requires medical attention.

Gallbladder series (GB series). A series of X-ray studies of the gallbladder and related structures, to diagnose disorders in that part of the body. *See also* Digestive system.

Gamma globulin. Immunoglobulin protein fractions in the blood that are antibodies. Given by injection, gamma globulin prevents or reduces the severity of infections such as German measles, measles, or hepatitis. *See also* Immunoglobulin.

Ganglion. A spongy collection of tissue that may form a cyst, usually on the wrist or the upper surface of the foot. As the ganglion grows, it may press on sensitive nerves in the affected area. Other symptoms include swelling, pain, numbness, or tingling. Treatment usually involves removal of the cyst by surgery.

Gardnerella. An organism often present in the vagina without causing disease. Some women with very large numbers of gardnerella develop an infection that may be sexually transmitted.

If Gardnerella infection occurs, you need to know the following:
Cause: The bacteria *Gardnerella (Hemophilus) vaginalis.*

Symptoms: Sometimes none; sometimes itching and a grayish-white discharge with an unpleasant odor.
Transmission: Gardnerella may sometimes be spread during sexual activity.
Treatment: Several types of antibiotics can cure gardnerella infection. If the infection returns after treatment, the sex partner must also be treated.
Complications: Scratching may cause a secondary infection.
Special precautions: No sex until a doctor confirms that the infection has been cleared up.

Gastroenteritis. Inflammation of the intestinal tract, the food tube that extends from the mouth to the rectum. Gastroenteritis may be caused by infection, various diseases, and certain drugs that irritate the intestinal lining. *See also* Digestive system.

Gastrointestinal series (GI series). A series of X-ray studies of the esophagus, stomach, and small bowel. An upper GI series includes just the esophagus, stomach, and duodenum (the first part of the intestine). The patient drinks a barium solution to make the organs more visible. During the next several hours, as the barium moves through the intestinal tract, X rays are taken at intervals. These help the physician to diagnose any problems in these areas. *See also* Digestive system.

Gastroscopy. Examination of the stomach with a gastroscope, an instrument that is passed through the mouth, through the food tube, and into the stomach to allow a doctor to examine it for abnormalities. *See also* Endoscopy.

Gay. Slang term used to describe a person (male or female) who is sexually attracted to others of the same sex.

Gay bowel disease. Certain infections and

other bowel problems sometimes diagnosed in men who have unprotected anal sex with other men.

Genes. Tiny units in living cells that carry traits inherited from parents. *See also* Chromosome.

Genetic counseling. A service provided by a specialist in this field, primarily to advise health professionals and the public about how certain characteristics and disease traits are transmitted from parents to children. Couples learn their chances of transmitting inheritable traits found in one or both partners' family backgrounds to a prospective child, so they can make an informed decision about having a child.

Genetics. A branch of medical science devoted to the study of inherited traits, conditions, and diseases, carried out by specialists (geneticists) who research these conditions, analyze them, and advise health professionals and patients concerning their conditions.

Genital, genitalia. The male and female organs of reproduction. In females these include the vagina, vulva (outer portion of the vagina), uterus (womb), fallopian tubes, and ovaries. In males they include the penis, testicles, and prostate gland. *See also* Reproductive system, female; male.

Genital hygiene. Methods used to keep the external genitalia (penis, vagina) clean and healthy.

Genital warts (HPV). A sexually transmitted disease, scientific name: *Condylomata acuminata*. Each year three to four million new cases of HPV infection are diagnosed in young people.
> *Cause:* The human papilloma virus (HPV).
> *Symptoms:* Genital warts are brown, pink, or dark gray. They are usually located in the moist areas of the male and female genitals or rectum. Warts appear singly or, more often, in a cluster that resembles a cauliflower. They may lie flat on the skin or sit on a small stalk. They bleed when hit or scratched.
> *Transmission:* Spread by an infected person to a healthy partner during sexual contact.
> *Treatment:* Removal of the warts by one of the following methods, depending on the location and number of warts found:
> * Caustic liquids (podophyllin or trichloroacetic acid)
> * Freezing agents (liquid nitrogen)
> * Electric cautery to burn off the lesions
> * Laser therapy; an intense beam of light is aimed at the lesion to destroy it.
>
> A person with genital warts should wear loose-fitting clothing and avoid tight underwear and jeans so that air can circulate and keep the treated area dry.
> *Complications:* Bleeding; secondary infection caused by scratching itchy lesions; cancer of the genitals, caused by certain HPV subtypes.
> *Special precautions:* No sex until a doctor or other health professional confirms that treatment has been successful. **Very important:** A condom must be worn even after the warts have been treated and destroyed. The warts may return and may be infectious even before they are visible.

Genitourinary (GU) tract. The external genitals, the internal genitals, and the urinary tract.

In females the external genitals include the vulva and the vagina. In males they include the penis, scrotum, and testicles.

In females the internal reproductive organs consist of the cervix, uterus, fallopian tubes, and ovaries; in males they include the prostate gland, epididymis, vas deferens, and seminal vesicles.

The urinary tract consists of two ureters (long tubes, each attached to a kidney at one end and the urinary bladder at the other); the urinary bladder; and the urethra, a tube that runs from the bladder to the tip of the penis in males and to an opening above the vagina in females.

The ureters carry urine produced in the kidneys to the bladder for storage. During urination, the urine is released from the bladder, flows through the urethra, and exits from the body.

German measles. *See* Measles, German.

Gingivitis. Inflammation of the gums. May be caused by irritating foods, infection, or certain diseases.

Gland. An organ that produces chemicals used in the body. There are two kinds of glands:
Endocrine glands, which discharge chemicals directly into the bloodstream—for example, the pituitary gland, located in the brain.
Exocrine glands, which discharge chemicals through tiny tubes (ducts) to nearby areas—for example, the salivary glands, located in the mouth.
See also Endocrine gland, Exocrine gland.

Glans. The tip, or head, of the penis.

Glaucoma. A condition in which the fluid pressure inside the eye is increased. Glaucoma is very dangerous. It must be treated promptly by a doctor or blindness may result. *See also* Intraocular pressure.

Glucose tolerance test (GTT). A test to find out if the body is using (metabolizing) blood sugar (glucose) normally. The patient either drinks glucose (oral glucose tolerance test) or receives an intravenous injection of glucose (intravenous glucose tolerance test). Blood is then drawn at hourly intervals to measure blood sugar levels. This test is often used to diagnose diabetes mellitus or to monitor blood sugar levels in a patient being

treated for diabetes. *See also* Diabetes mellitus.

Gonad. Reproductive or sex gland. In the male, the testis; in the female, the ovary. *See also* Endocrine gland.

Gonadotropins. Hormones secreted by the pituitary gland located in the brain. These hormones stimulate the growth and development of the sex glands.

Gonorrhea. A sexually transmitted disease.
Cause: The gonococcus organism (*Neisseria gonorrhoeae*).
Symptoms in men:
• Inflammation of the urinary tube (urethra)
• Discharge from the penis (watery, then pus-filled)
• Frequent urinating; may be painful
• Reddened area around the urinary opening at the tip of the penis
• Swollen glands in the groin
Symptoms in women:
• Inflammation of the urinary tube (urethra) and the cervix
• Cervical discharge
• Pain when urinating
• Uncomfortable feeling in the lower abdomen
• A reddened, swollen cervix, found on internal examination
• Excessive bleeding during or between periods
Symptoms in men and women:
• Sore throat; may develop if an infected person's genitals come in contact with the sex partner's mouth
• Inflamed rectum; may develop if an infected person's genitals come in contact with the sex partner's rectum
Symptoms in girls before puberty:
• Frequent urinating
• Inflammation of the vagina that causes itching, and a pus-filled vaginal discharge

Symptoms in newborn infants:
- Eye infection may develop after the baby passes through the infected mother's birth canal during delivery

Treatment: Prompt treatment with powerful antibiotic drugs will cure this infection. Early diagnosis and treatment are essential to avoid infecting others and to prevent serious complications.

Complications in men:
- Pain and swelling in the groin and testicles
- Chills and fever
- Arthritis

Complications in women:
- Acute pelvic inflammatory disease (PID), which involves severe inflammation of the entire external and internal female reproductive tract, often with a high fever and severe abdominal pain. Acute PID may require hospitalization for treatment and to prevent even more serious, sometimes life-threatening, complications. These include:
  - Chronic pain
  - Scar tissue in the fallopian tubes
  - Pregnancy in a fallopian tube instead of in the uterus
  - Infertility
  - Arthritis

Complications in men and women:
- Pain and swelling in the joints of the fingers, wrists, knees, ankles, and toes
- Rash on the hands, feet, ankles, and toes

Special precautions: No sexual activity or contact until a doctor confirms that the infection has been cured.

Gossypol. An experimental birth control pill for men. Made from cottonseed, this pill prevents production of sperm in the testicles. It may sometimes result in permanent sterility. It is not available for general use at this time. *See also* Contraceptive.

Grafenberg spot (G spot). An area deep inside the vagina. The G spot may be associated with sexual stimulation and pleasure. A controversy exists about the G spot: some claim it exists, others that it doesn't.

Grippe. *See* Flu.

Growth curves. The two charts of growth curves, one for females and one for males, show the normal range of height and weight for young Americans as compiled by the National Center for Health Statistics. The curved lines for height and for weight represent percentiles, or statistical measurements, based on one hundred individuals.

Using growth curves, female and male

To place an individual within these scales, find the age at the bottom of the chart and the height (in inches or centimeters) along the left side of the chart. Draw a line up from the age, and a line out from the height column. Where the two lines meet indicates the person's percentile ranking. As an example, a fourteen-year-old girl who is 60 inches tall is in the 10th percentile for height. (Out of 100 girls, 90 will be taller, 9 will be shorter). *See also* page 58.

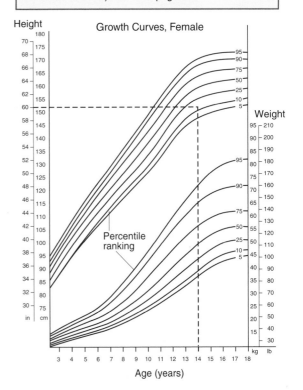

Growth Curves, Female

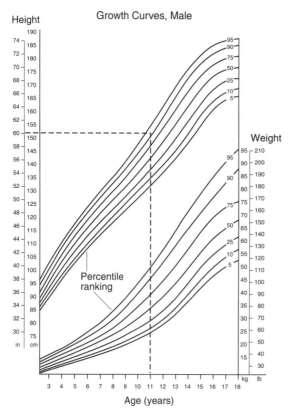

Growth Curves, Male

Height

Weight

Percentile ranking

Age (years)

Growth hormone: human growth hormone (HGH). A hormone secreted by the pituitary gland. The hormone stimulates body growth and has other functions.

Gynecological (pelvic) examination. Adult women should have annual gynecological examinations. Teenagers who are sexually active should also have exams. Moderate to frequent sexual activity, especially with multiple partners, increases the risk of STDs and cervical cancer for teens.

Gynecology. The medical specialty that deals with the study and treatment of diseases and abnormalities and the normal functions of a female's reproductive organs.

Gynecomastia. Enlargement of the breasts in males. In a teenage boy this may be a temporary condition of no significance. However, enlarged breasts may indicate a health problem. A medical examination is necessary.

H

Hair loss (baldness). The thinning, or disappearance of hair on a person's head. In a teenage person, the hair of the head may become thin or fall out as a result of a fever, certain medications such as chemotherapy given for certain cancers, or a skin condition such as ringworm. These conditions are usually temporary, and the hair regrows once the condition is improved, or the medication is discontinued. Some people lose hair after trying to straighten, curl, or otherwise manipulate their hair, which may cause damage. Stress, hormonal changes, and autoimmune disorders may also cause hair loss (alopecia).

Hair, pubic. Hair that begins to grow around the genitals during adolescence. The first few hairs appear between the ages of eight and fourteen. Initially thin and straight, pubic hair gradually becomes thicker and curly. As a teen grows older, pubic hair grows in a triangular adult pattern. *See also* Tanner stages.

Hair, underarm. Hair that appears in the armpits at age twelve to fourteen.

Halitosis. *See* Bad breath.

Hallucination. An inaccurate perception of the senses; something seen or felt or heard that isn't there. Hallucinations may be a symptom of mental illness or they may occur after taking certain drugs or chemicals. They may also accompany some physical illnesses.

Hard-on. *See* Erection; Tumescence.

Headache. A pain in the head. Headaches occur because of tension, fatigue, stress, fever, drinking alcohol, certain drugs, and for various other reasons. Over-the-counter pain relievers are often effective. Frequent, severe, or long-lasting headaches should be re-ported to a doctor, especially if accompanied by nausea, vomiting, or vision changes. *See also* Migraine; Tension headache.

Health risks. You take risks that may affect your health if you:

- Get too little sleep
- Eat too much and gain excessive weight
- Eat too little, and lose more weight than is healthy, or eat a poorly balanced diet
- Get too little regular exercise (A teen "couch potato" usually has poor muscle tone and poor blood circulation, which can lead to other complications.)

Other serious health risks threaten teen-agers who:

- Smoke
- Drink alcohol
- Use drugs other than those suggested or prescribed by a health professional
- Drive after using alcohol or drugs
- Expose themselves to AIDS and other sexually transmitted diseases by having sex with an infected partner,
- Expose themselves to AIDS by sharing needles and other equipment that may nick or cut their skin, allowing HIV, the AIDS virus, to enter the bloodstream and cause HIV infection and AIDS

Hearing loss. *See* Deafness.

Hearing test. *See* Audiogram.

Heart. A muscular organ in the chest. The heart is a strong, life-essential organ with two separate major functions. (1) Right heart: to pump deoxygenated (used) blood into the lungs where it receives new oxygen. (2) Left heart: to pump freshly oxygenated blood into the major arteries and throughout the body to nourish all tissues. The heart keeps the circulation going so that blood cells will make the rounds of the circulatory system up to 5,000 times in twenty-four hours. *See also* Blood; Circulation.

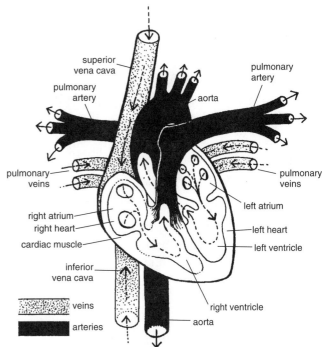

Note: The pulmonary artery carries deoxygenated blood from the right heart to the lungs. Pulmonary veins carry oxygenated blood from the lungs to the left heart.

Heart murmur. A heart sound. Health professionals can determine normal or abnormal heart functioning by listening for heart sounds with a stethoscope.

The "lub-dub" and other sounds heard through the stethoscope are made by valves inside the heart's chambers that click open and shut as blood passes in and out. Different sounds made by the valves indicate the quality of various heart functions. A murmur heard through the stethoscope does not necessarily mean something is wrong. Health professionals can tell the difference between a murmur that has no special significance and one that indicates a defect or illness.

Heart palpitations. *See* Palpitation.

Heatstroke. *See* Sunstroke.

Heimlich maneuver. A procedure used to dislodge food or other material caught in a person's throat and causing choking. This can happen if a person eats too fast, does not chew a portion of food thoroughly, or inhales while chewing. The food slips down the windpipe (trachea) instead of the gullet (esophagus). If it lodges in the trachea, little or no air gets into the lungs and the person begins to choke.

The Heimlich maneuver, named for the physician who developed it, has saved the lives of many choking people. For instructions on how to perform the procedure, *see* Appendix F: First Aid, Heimlich maneuver.

Hematocrit test (Hct). A measure of the volume of red blood cells in whole blood. Red blood cells are one component of whole blood.

Hematoma. Bleeding somewhere inside the body. The blood collects and forms a clot. A hematoma occurs after trauma or a blow on some part of the body, which starts the bleeding.

A small hematoma may resolve by itself. A larger hematoma under the skin may be aspirated with a syringe and needle, to remove the blood. A large hematoma deep inside the body may need to be evacuated by surgery.

Hemodialysis. *See* Kidneys.

Hemoglobin (Hb, Hgb). A protein pigment in the blood that carries oxygen and carbon dioxide. *See also* Blood.

Hemoglobin, glycosylated (HbA$_{1c}$). A type of hemoglobin present in a higher percentage in a person who has elevated blood sugar levels, such as someone who has diabetes mellitus. Measurement of this hemoglobin determines blood sugar content over a period of time, an indication of how well a diabetic patient is responding to treatment. The treatment (insulin dosage) is then modified as needed. *See also* Diabetes mellitus.

Hemophilia. A hereditary illness seen almost exclusively in males. A person with he-

mophilia lacks essential blood factors that help the blood to clot. As a result, the blood clots very slowly after a cut or surgery, often causing prolonged bleeding or hemorrhage (severe bleeding). A transfusion of the missing blood factors helps to stop the bleeding and to prevent other bleeding incidents. Unfortunately, many hemophiliacs have developed HIV infection and AIDS due to HIV-contaminated transfusions of clotting factors. Most of these infections occurred before a test for HIV was available to blood banks. Today, all blood is tested before being used for transfusions, and contaminated or infected blood is discarded.

Hemorrhoids. Enlarged veins, usually found around or inside the rectum. Hemorrhoids may itch, hurt, and bleed, especially when a person is constipated.

A doctor can suggest several effective treatments; the choice depends on the amount of bleeding and the extent of discomfort. Anyone who notices rectal bleeding needs to be examined to determine if the cause is hemorrhoids or a more serious illness.

Hepatitis. Inflammation of the liver that may, in some cases, lead to destruction of the organ.

Cause: Various drugs, toxins, chemicals, and infections, and certain viruses, including the hepatitis A, B, C, D, and E viruses.

Transmission: There are differences in the means of transmission and the extent of the liver damage caused by each of these viruses. The viruses can be passed through contaminated food or water, through saliva, unprotected sexual relations with an infected person, sharing of contaminated needles, and breast milk from an infected mother.

Symptoms: Abdominal pain, jaundice (yellow skin), dark urine, enlargement of the liver, lack of appetite, nausea and vomiting, fever, and severe fatigue.

Treatment: There is no specific treatment for most types of hepatitis. Doctors usually prescribe rest and frequent small, nutritious meals.

Fortunately, the liver is an organ that can repair itself; many people recover completely from the illness within a few weeks. Some, however, remain contagious for many years. A few may suffer such extensive liver damage that repair is not possible and the patient dies.

Special precautions: No one should have unprotected sex with a person who has, or may have hepatitis. Any person in contact with someone who has active hepatitis A or B infection should receive a protective injection of immunoglobulin (*see* Immunoglobulin) to avoid contracting the disease. And those likely to be in frequent contact with persons who have hepatitis B—for example, health care personnel—should receive immunization with hepatitis B vaccine (Engerix B, Recombivax). Infants are now routinely vaccinated against hepatitis B. Teens and young adults should ask their doctors about the vaccine during routine health visits, as a series of three injections can prevent this very serious illness. A vaccine against Hepatitis A is now available; at this time there is none against the other types of viral hepatitis.

Hepatitis screen. A blood test to detect different types of hepatitis, usually hepatitis A, B, or C. *See also* Hepatitis.

Hepatosplenomegaly. Enlargement of the liver and spleen, a symptom in a number of diseases (hepato means liver; spleno, spleen; megaly, enlargement).

Herbalism. Treatments intended to prevent, cure, or relieve conditions with the use of natural substances such as plants (leaves, flowers, bark, seeds, roots). The substances may be used as they are found, or brewed as a tea, mixed with other substances, as liquids, ointments, or in pills.

Hermaphrodite. A person born with both male and female sexual organs. A hermaphrodite does not have fully developed sex organs. During infancy, the baby's parents and doctor usually make the decision as to the sex in which the child will be raised. Surgery may be performed, as needed.

Hernia. A condition in which a body part or organ breaks through the surrounding muscular wall due to weakened muscles that are unable to hold the organ in place.

An intestinal hernia (a portion of intestine that has broken through a weakened part of the surrounding abdominal muscles) may cause pain in the groin and a bulge in the lower abdomen at the breakthrough site. If this portion of intestine is squeezed and becomes trapped inside the muscular wall, it may be deprived of its essential blood supply. This dangerous complication requires

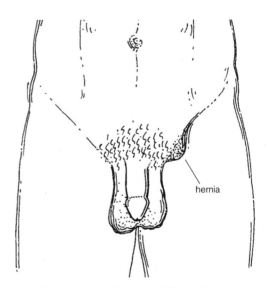

A hernia commonly occurs in the groin area.

prompt surgery to prevent tissue death and to restore a firm muscular wall.

Heroin. A street drug. *See* Appendix C: Street drugs.

Herpes infection. A common virus infection that may affect the eyes, lips, or fingers. Herpes infection also occurs in the genital area and nearby areas.

Cause: Herpes simplex virus. There are two main types: herpes simplex virus type 1 (HSV-1) and herpes simplex virus type 2 (HSV-2). Both types of HSV may cause infection.

Transmission in the upper part of the body: Contact with an infected person's lesions, contaminated towels, or other infected materials.

Transmission in the genital area: Almost always through unprotected oral or genital contact with an infected partner.

Symptoms: Redness and small blisters on and around the affected areas. Itching and burning may be felt before there are any visible signs. The blisters may itch, burn, and discharge fluid. Visible herpes lesions and discharges usually last about five days and are highly infectious.

Once herpes-virus infection is established in the body, the virus can travel to nearby nerves, where it remains for life, even after lesions have healed and are no longer visible. From time to time, the virus may become active again, causing new (recurrent) bouts of infection.

Shedding the herpes virus: A person who has had a bout of genital herpes infection may shed (discharge) herpes virus. Viral shedding may occur following the first bout, or before new lesions appear in a recurrence. A healthy person who has sex with a herpes-shedding partner may contract genital herpes-virus infection.

Treatment: The drug Zovirax helps to heal the blisters, relieves pain and itching, and controls but does not cure the infection. Several other medications are available for recurring bouts of infection.

Complications: A secondary bacterial infection may develop at the blister sites due to scratching. The infection may also spread to other body areas.

Special precautions: A person with genital herpes infection should not have sex while blisters are present in the genital area. A medical examination is needed to confirm that all lesions have healed and that sexual activities may be resumed safely, provided that condoms are used.

Herpes zoster (shingles). *See* Shingles.

Heterophil agglutination test. A blood test used to detect acute infectious mononucleosis. *See also* Mononucleosis.

Heterosexuality. Sexual attraction to persons of the opposite sex.

High blood pressure. *See* Hypertension.

High density lipoprotein cholesterol (HDLC). *See* Cholesterol profile.

High-risk behavior. Any behavior or action likely to cause illness or harm. *See also* Health risks.

Hip pointer. A sports injury that causes painful bruising on the upper part of the hipbone. *See also* Sports injuries.

Hirsutism. Excessive growth of body hair in women, usually caused by a glandular condition.

Hives, urticaria. An allergic skin condition that appears as itchy red blotches or welts. A doctor can determine the cause of the allergy and prescribe an antiallergenic drug to treat it and eliminate the hives.

HIV (HIV-1, HIV-2). Human immunodeficiency virus, the virus that causes HIV infection and AIDS. HIV-1 causes most cases of HIV infection and AIDS. HIV-2 also causes this infection, but is rarely seen in the United States. *See also* AIDS; ELISA.

HIV infection. *See* AIDS.

HIV tests. Laboratory procedures to determine if HIV or HIV antibodies are present in blood. *See also* AIDS.

Hodgkin's disease. A cancerous disease of the lymph glands that occurs often in young people. A person with Hodgkin's disease develops one or more swollen lymph glands, often in the neck, the armpit, or the groin. Other symptoms include weakness, sweating, fever, weight loss, and constant tiredness.

Hodgkin's disease has a very high cure rate if it is discovered early and treated promptly. Treatment consists of radiation therapy and chemotherapy. A patient who becomes resistant to treatment, whose disease is far advanced, or who has frequent recurrences of disease, may require additional treatment, such as a bone marrow transplant or a transfusion of certain blood cells given by plasmapheresis. This process involves taking blood from the patient and removing specific blood cells by spinning the blood at high speed in the laboratory (centrifugation). The blood is then returned to the patient.

A patient who has recovered from Hodgkin's disease must have periodic checkups to be sure the disease has not recurred, or, if it has, to receive further treatment.

Holistic health care. Treatment centered on the complete person, not just the diseased body part. The holistic health care practitioner examines and treats the physical problem, and also checks for other problems, due to emotional or other concerns, or caused by the patient's lifestyle, that may affect the physical problem. All of these problems are then addressed at the same time to achieve relief and a cure.

There are many types of holistic (alternative) health care methods. These include acupuncture, herbalism, homeopathy, naturopathy, and chiropractic. *See also* these entries.

Homeopathy. A treatment in which very small amounts of medications are given to produce symptoms similar to those of the complaint being treated, but much milder. The assumption is that the body can cope with a small quantity of an irritating substance, and may so develop the ability to overcome the problem.

Homosexuality. Sexual attraction to persons of the same sex.

Hormones. Chemical substances produced naturally by various endocrine glands and discharged into the bloodstream. They are carried to various organs and body systems that need them to function normally. *See also* Gland.

Human chorionic gonadotropin (HCG). A hormone present in the placenta, the sac surrounding the growing fetus in the mother's womb. High levels of this hormone, when found in a woman's blood, usually indicate that she is pregnant. Elevated HCG in a nonpregnant woman's blood indicates a problem in the reproductive system. *See also* Pregnancy test.

Human growth hormone (HGH). *See* Growth hormone.

Human immunodeficiency virus (HIV). *See* HIV; AIDS.

Human papillomavirus (HPV). *See* Genital warts.

Hydrocele. A swelling inside the scrotum, caused by a collection of fluid in the scrotal sac that surrounds the testicle. Fluid may collect as a result of inflammation or a hernia. A doctor needs to examine the scrotum if there

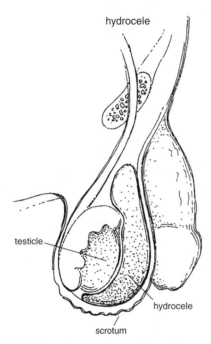

If fluid collects between the testicle and its covering, a hydrocele forms.

is pain or considerable swelling, to determine if treatment is required. Surgery can correct this condition.

Hymen. A thin tissue (membrane) covering the vaginal opening in young girls. The hymen may stretch, be pulled to one side, or even disappear as a result of a medical examination, sexual intercourse, or injury. *See also* Imperforate hymen.

Hyperactivity. Excessive display of energy, and sometimes, aggression. Children are born with a wide range of temperaments. Some children are active, full of energy and ambition. Others are less active, even sluggish, with a minimum of energy. Still others are hyperactive, with excessive energy, which may be coupled with aggressive behavior and inability to pay attention for any length of time. Severe hyperactivity, with excessive energy and inattention, is called attention deficit disorder (ADD). *See* ADD.

Hypermetropia. *See* Eye disorders.

Hypertension (HTN, HBP). High blood pressure that occurs as a result of the action of certain body chemicals, or when fatty lumps (plaques) are deposited on the inner surface of blood vessel walls. Plaques narrow the space needed for effective blood flow.

Constant elevated pressure of blood against the plaque-narrowed blood vessels causes further damage and may block essential blood flow to certain body areas. When that happens, nearby tissues die due to lack of nourishment. Serious illness may result. If one of the main blood vessels of the heart is starved and becomes narrowed or shut off, a heart attack results.

Prevention: Exercise and a healthy, low-fat diet help to prevent high blood pressure.

Treatment: High blood pressure can often be lowered by a program of prescribed exercises and by changing the diet. Drugs are available to treat high blood pressure if diet and exercise are not effective.

Hyperventilation. Excessive breathing (respiration). People with great anxiety may hyperventilate (breathe in and out too rapidly), claiming they "can't get enough air." In fact, they may overbreathe as a result of their anxiety. If the overbreathing persists for some time, it may cause chemical changes in the blood.

Excessive respirations cause a loss of carbon dioxide and an excessive intake of oxygen. The result may be lightheadedness, even fainting. Other symptoms of hyperventilation may include numbness or tingling in the lips or hands. These complaints may progress to spasms of the hands and feet. Some people may think they are having a heart problem. Asthma, some other respiratory illnesses, and other conditions, may also cause hyperventilation.

The diagnosis is made by physical examinations and blood tests. If hyperventilation is found to be due to anxiety, reassurance and counseling may help the patient overcome the problem. During an acute episode, breathing into a paper bag, which conserves exhaled carbon monoxide, may be helpful.

Hyphema. A collection of blood in the clear anterior (forward) chamber of the eye following a blow to that area. Treatment includes bed rest and observation. Further measures may be needed if the condition worsens.

Hypochondria. A mental state in which a healthy person believes he or she is ill. Some people develop hypochondria because they are very anxious about their health or other matters in their lives. They are convinced that they have symptoms of illnesses, even when a medical examination shows them to be healthy. Counseling or psychological treatment may be needed to help a hypochondriacal person.

Hypoglycemia. Very low blood sugar content. Effects—especially in diabetic patients receiving insulin—include hunger, weakness, sweating, and other symptoms. Sugar in the form of fruit or candy may relieve the symptoms. Food intake and insulin dosage may need to be modified. *See also* Diabetes mellitus.

Hypospadias. A birth defect in which the urinary tube is incomplete and opens on the underside of the penis. Surgery is usually required to repair the defect.

Hypothalamic pituitary adrenal axis (HPA axis). Refers to interactive functions of the hypothalamus, pituitary, and adrenal glands. The hypothalamus controls release of hormones to the pituitary gland, which releases still other hormones into the blood. These hormones are secreted by the ovary, thyroid, and adrenal glands. Together, they control many body functions.

I

Icteric. Yellow, jaundiced. Icteric skin and eyes are yellowish, a result of gallbladder or liver disease, or due to destruction of red blood cells.

Icterus. Jaundice.

Idiopathic thrombocytopenic purpura (ITP). *See* Thrombocytopenic purpura.

Ileostomy. *See* Ostomy.

Immune booster. A repeat injection, usually given several years later, of a vaccine to strengthen and maintain protection against infectious diseases such as measles or whooping cough. *See also* Immunization.

Immune system. The body's defense against infection and other harmful substances. It employs substances called antibodies that are produced in the bone marrow, the thymus gland, and the lymph glands. Antibodies make up the defense team that fights infection and agents that may harm the body.

Immunization. A process, achieved in one of several ways, of protecting a person against various diseases or infections. There are two methods of immunization: active immunization and passive immunization.

Active immunization involves injection of a vaccine containing a small amount of an infectious agent that has been killed or modified (inactivated). The injection does not cause illness, but allows the person's immune system to produce his or her own antibodies, which then protect against the disease, usually for life. This process of stimulating antibodies requires a period of weeks or months. For this reason, active immunization must be

Recommended immunization schedule for teens and preteens		
Age	Vaccine	Method
11–12 years	Measles (M)	Injection
	Mumps (M)	Injection
	Rubella (R)	Injection
14–16 years	Diphtheria	Injection
	Tetanus	Injection
	MMR (if not given earlier)	Injection
	Varivax (2 doses, 4–8 weeks apart; if not given earlier and if no exposure to chicken pox)	Injection
	Hepatitis B (3 separate doses; if not given earlier)	Injection
Annually	PPD (purified protein derivative, to test for TB exposure)	Injection
	Flu shots (for teens with chronic illness and those who smoke)	Injection

used as a prophylactic (preventive) procedure that is given some time before exposure to an infection.

Vaccines are given by injection, except for polio vaccine, which can be given by mouth or by injection. Vaccines are available for the following diseases: hepatitis A and B, diphtheria, whooping cough (pertussis), tetanus, measles (rubeola), German measles (rubella), and mumps. Vaccination against these diseases should be started shortly after birth, and continued according to a prescribed schedule.

Passive immunization is a process used for people exposed to an infection for the first time. It consists of an injection of antibodies to a specific infection. The antibodies are derived from persons who have had the infection, and are then grown in a laboratory for use in other people. Passive immunization confers partial or complete protection against a specific infection for a short time, usually about two weeks. *See also* Gamma globulin.

Immunocompetence. The body's ability to defend itself against harmful substances and organisms. *See also* Immune system.

Immunodeficiency. Inability of the body to defend itself against harmful substances and organisms. Immunodeficiency may be due to weakness of the immune system, which cannot produce sufficient antibodies as a result of infection or abnormalities. Immunodeficiency may also be caused by a disorder of the immune system itself. Some causes of immunodeficiency are diseases such as AIDS, and medications used to treat certain types of cancer. Immunodeficiency is sometimes induced to prevent rejection of an organ transplant. Depending on the cause, immune deficiency may be temporary, and normal immune capacity returns. In other severe or progressive diseases, or in case of an inherited form of immunodeficiency, it may be long lasting or permanent. *See also* Immune system.

Immunoglobulin (IG). A group of body proteins that contain antibodies that fight specific infections. Given by injection, an immunoglobulin can protect a person exposed to an infection such as hepatitis, or lessen the severity of the infection.

Immunotherapy. Treatment to increase or strengthen a person's defenses against infection or disease. *See also* Immune system.

Imperforate hymen. Sometimes the hymen, a membrane that covers a girl's vagina during childhood, remains in place even after a girl starts to have menstrual periods. (Imperforate means having no opening.) With an intact hymen, menstrual blood cannot be discharged from the vagina. Instead, it backs up into the abdomen, causing pain and swelling. The girl may not be aware that she has begun to have periods, since she has not had any menstrual flow. A medical examination is needed to diagnose the problem. Treatment consists of surgery to remove the hymen. *See also* Hymen.

Impetigo. A skin infection caused by the staphylococcus or streptococcus organism. It is most often diagnosed in babies and small children. Impetigo generally appears on the face, arms, and legs. Reddened areas develop into blisters that are later covered with crusts. Impetigo is a highly contagious infection. It is treated with antibiotics.

Impotence. A male's inability to have an erection. Many factors can cause impotence. Psychological causes include anxiety, depression, and fear of failure during sexual intercourse. Physical causes include use of drugs or alcohol, certain medications prescribed for high blood pressure and other conditions, and circulatory problems that affect the blood supply to the penis.

Incest. Sexual intercourse between two close relatives—for example, a sister and brother or a father and son or daughter. Any child or teen who is forced to have sex with another family member needs to confide in an adult who can help to end this harmful situation.

Incubation period (IC). The time that elapses between being exposed to and becoming infected with a disease, and the appearance of the first symptoms. Infectious diseases have a wide range of incubation periods. The incubation period of the common cold and the more serious influenza (flu) is only one to three days; the IC of infectious mononucleosis is five to fifteen days, and that of chicken pox, two to three weeks. Generally speaking, an infectious disease is not transmitted to others during the incubation period.

Infatuation. Excessive interest, admiration, or love for another person.

Infection. A condition that arises when harmful organisms invade body cells and tissues, causing illness, destruction of tissues, and other harmful effects. Many infections can be transmitted to others in various ways: by touch, by sexual contact, through the air, through exposure to contaminated blood products (by transfusion or use of dirty needles), by eating or drinking contaminated food or fluids.

Infectious mononucleosis. *See* Mononucleosis.

Infertility. Inability to become pregnant or to cause a pregnancy. Infertility has many causes. In women the cause may be infection, disease, or abnormal development of the reproductive organs. In men, the causes include infection, disease, and abnormal development of the sperm-forming organs, resulting in poor sperm quality. A fertility specialist can often diagnose the cause and treat infertile people, allowing men and women to become fertile and have children.

Inflammation. A reaction by body tissues to damage caused by an injury or disease. Inflamed tissues become red, swollen, hot, and painful. Inflammation may occur in most parts of the body. Treatment depends on the cause of the inflammation, and the body area that is affected.

Inflammatory bowel disease. A chronic (long-term) disease of the lower bowel (intestine) of unknown causes.

Symptoms: Inflammation in different areas of the bowel, pain, cramps, diarrhea, fever, damage to the bowel wall such as ulcers.

Treatment: Determined by the location of the inflammation (either in the small intestine, Crohn's disease; or in the large bowel, ulcerative colitis) and its severity. Drugs control diarrhea. Steroid drugs and antibiotics reduce inflammation and eliminate infection. In severe cases a badly damaged section of bowel is removed, which often allows the patient to return to a normal life.

See also Crohn's disease; Ulcerative colitis.

Influenza. *See* Flu.

Ingrown toenail. A toenail, usually of a big toe, that grows inward toward the toe. An ingrown toenail may develop naturally, but more often it is caused by incorrect nail clipping, or by shoes that don't fit well. A badly ingrown toenail is painful, and the toe may become inflamed or infected. It generally needs medical attention from a doctor or a foot specialist (podiatrist).

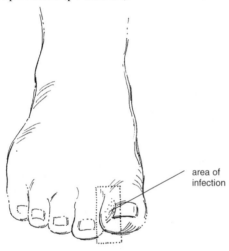

area of infection

Insomnia. Inability to sleep. May be caused by poor sleeping habits, excessive use of caffeine (coffee), lack of exercise, illness, stress or worry, or drug abuse. A healthy person who suffers from insomnia can overcome this problem by going to bed at a reasonable time every night; avoiding stimulating activities, foods, or drinks late in the evening; exercising regularly; and not napping during the day.

A person who is ill may be given a prescription for a sleeping medication, but should stop using it as soon as he or she feels better, to avoid becoming dependent on the drug.

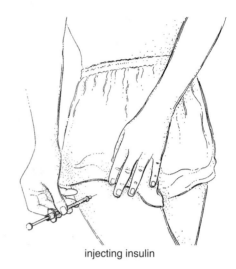

injecting insulin

Insulin. A hormone produced by the pancreas gland. Insulin is essential in the body's regulation (metabolism) of carbohydrates (sugars and starches). A person whose body does not produce enough insulin, or cannot use insulin adequately, may develop diabetes. *See also* Diabetes mellitus.

Insulin as a treatment for diabetes: Synthetically produced (from a human gene) or made from animal (beef, pork) tissue, insulin is used to treat children, teens, and adults to control their diabetes. Prescribed amounts of insulin, along with a special diet, will keep the disease under control. There is no cure at this time. A person who requires insulin must take insulin by injection once or more often every day.

Tests to check blood sugar: The diabetic person must test his or her blood at regular intervals to see if the insulin dosage is keeping the blood sugar level at a normal or near normal level. If not, a doctor adjusts the insulin dosage.

Insulin-dependent diabetes mellitus (IDDM). *See* Diabetes mellitus.

Intake and output (I&O). The amount of liquid taken in and eliminated by the body. Measurement of intake and output helps the doctor to determine if a person, often a hospitalized patient, is receiving enough fluid for normal body functioning.

Intercourse, sexual. Sexual contact between two partners. There are various kinds of sexual contact:

Genital intercourse: A sexual act involving insertion of the man's penis in the woman's vagina.

Oral sex: A sexual act in which one partner's mouth is in contact with the other partner's genitals. Fellatio is contact between one person's mouth and a partner's penis; cunnilingus is contact between one person's mouth and a woman's vagina.

Anal sex: A sexual act in which a man inserts his penis in the rectum of his sex partner.

Intestine. A portion of the digestive tract that begins at the stomach and ends at the rectum. The intestine has two parts.

The small intestine (about 22 feet long), receives partly digested food from the stomach. The food is digested further by enzymes and other juices coming from the liver, gallbladder, and pancreas. Muscular contractions move the food along the intestinal tract, and nutrients are absorbed by blood vessels and carried to the liver for storage.

The large intestine (colon) reabsorbs most of the digestive fluid. The remaining solid waste is transported to the rectum, where it is eliminated in bowel movements (feces). *See also* Digestion; Digestive system.

Intimacy. Feelings of closeness and deep understanding between people. The term may also be used to mean sexual activity.

Intramuscular (IM). Administered by injection (of a prescribed drug) into the muscular tissue of the upper arm, hip, or buttock.

Intraocular pressure (IOP). The pressure inside the eyeball. Increased pressure in the eye may cause a dangerous condition called glaucoma. If glaucoma is not treated, it may cause loss of vision. Eye doctors routinely measure intraocular pressure when they check a person's eyes.

Intrauterine device (IUD). A small metal or plastic device inserted into a woman's uterus (womb) to prevent pregnancy. *See also* Contraceptive.

Insertion of an IUD: A doctor or other health professional performs a pelvic examination to make sure there is no infection or other condition that would make IUD use undesirable or harmful, and then inserts the device.

How the IUD works: After insertion, the IUD is left in place for a year or longer. It works in one of several ways: It may prevent sperm from traveling to the fallopian tube to fertilize the egg, it may prevent fertilization itself, or it may interfere with the implanting of the egg by making the uterine lining too thin to allow the egg to settle in and develop.

Some women may experience more bleeding than usual, and some may have

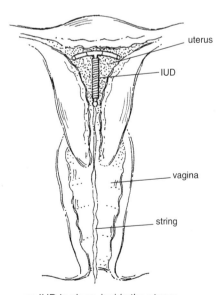

an IUD in place, inside the uterus

pain or other complications. If these symptoms persist, the IUD may have to be removed. Occasionally, a woman's body may expel the IUD, which then needs to be replaced.

Effectiveness: The IUD is a very effective contraceptive device, with a high rate of pregnancy prevention.

Intravenous (IV). Intravenous means "into a vein" and refers to injecting a prescribed medication or liquid directly into a vein. It is also used to refer to street drugs injected into a vein.

Intravenous drug (IV drug). A drug injected into a vein. An intravenous drug takes effect much more rapidly than one taken by mouth. Speed is often important—for example, in emergency treatment, where every minute counts in saving a person's life. Drug abusers may use intravenous self-injection (shooting up) to achieve a quick high from a street drug.

Intravenous drug abuser (IV drug abuser, IVDA). A person who illegally obtains drugs for self-injection into a vein, to get high.

IV drug abusers expose themselves to serious health risks. They may become addicted to the drug or substance, requiring more frequent injections and higher doses over time to get high. Many IV drug abusers lose control over their lives in a short time. They want more of the drug, and have to find (or steal) money to pay for it, in order to satisfy their craving.

Intravenous drug abusers often share dirty syringes and needles and may thus contract infections such as hepatitis or HIV infection.

Intravenous pyelogram (IVP). A test of kidney and urinary tract structure and function. Dye (contrast material) is injected into a vein in the arm or leg. X rays taken at intervals indicate how well the kidneys trans-

port urine to the bladder. It also shows abnormalities of the kidneys, ureters, and bladder.

In vitro fertilization (IVF). A process in which a woman's egg is removed from her ovary, and fertilized in a laboratory with sperm from her husband or a sperm donor. This procedure is sometimes used when a woman has been unable to become pregnant.

Irregular periods. Menstrual periods that don't occur in a regular pattern of every twenty-eight to thirty days. A girl's first few periods are often irregular, which is normal. If periods continue to be irregular, a medical examination is needed to check for health problems that require treatment. Overexercising and low body weight may lead to irregular periods. *See also* Menstruation.

Irritable bowel. A combination of intestinal discomfort, gas, and diarrhea that may occur from time to time. Irritable bowel may be genetic (other family members may also have it), it may occur after eating certain foods or using a particular drug, it may follow various infectious or other intestinal diseases, or it may indicate stress.

Isolation. Confinement of a person with an infectious disease in a separate room or other space away from other family members, or from other patients in the hospital, to prevent spread of the infection.

IUD. *See* Intrauterine device.

J

Jaundice. Yellowish-greenish discoloration of the skin and the whites of the eyes. This change in skin color is caused by a build-up of bile pigments (called bilirubin) in blood, due to an infection, or an illness, such as cancer, that affects the gallbladder, liver, or pancreas. For example, a tumor may obstruct the passage of bile from the gallbladder, bile duct, pancreas, or liver into the intestinal tract for elimination.

Newborn babies occasionally are somewhat jaundiced during the first few days of life, due to immaturity of the liver, and an increase of bile pigments in the blood. This condition usually clears up without treatment. If it persists, or if the bilirubin level is very high, the pediatrician will search for the specific cause of the problem.

Jaundice is a symptom, not a disease. Anyone who notices this symptom should immediately consult a physician, who will diagnose the cause and prescribe treatment.

Jelly, contraceptive. An over-the-counter, water-based substance that contains a sperm-killing (spermicidal) chemical. It is used alone, or together with a barrier contraceptive, such as a diaphragm or condom, to prevent pregnancy. *See also* Contraceptive.

Jock itch. An itchy, scaly, fungal infection that can affect a man's groin, the inner parts of the thighs, the scrotum, and sometimes the area around the rectum. The fungus that causes jock itch lives in warm, moist areas such as the groin.

Antifungal medication (*see* Appendix B, Antifungal medications), exposure of the affected area to air, and clean, loose-fitting underwear will cure the infection. Avoid wearing tight underclothes because they can chafe, allowing the fungus to penetrate the skin and cause further infection.

Jockstrap. A cloth support for male genitals, worn for comfort and protection.

Junk food. Food that has little or no nutritional value. Junk foods may taste good because they contain a lot of fat, sugar, or salt. A person who eats a lot of junk food often gains weight but gets few essential proteins, vitamins, and minerals, which are usually missing from these foods.

Juvenile rheumatoid arthritis (JRA). A form of arthritis that affects children and adolescents. The cause is unknown. Symptoms of JRA include pain, redness, stiffness, and swelling of the joints (wrists, elbows, hips, knees, and ankles).

There are several types of JRA, each with somewhat different symptoms. Symptoms may involve joints, the lymph nodes, and the eyes.

Treatment includes over-the-counter anti-inflammatory drugs. More potent medications such as steroids may be prescribed to control severe flare-ups of inflamed joints and other symptoms.

K

Kaposi's sarcoma. A cancerous growth on the skin and in internal organs, found mainly in people who have AIDS.

Keloid. A section of scar tissue that keeps growing, often into a large mass of tissue. Keloids may occur in the scar of a healing surgical incision, or following other skin injuries, including ear piercing.

A keloid is not dangerous, but may be unsightly. Treatment may consist of cortisone ointment or cream and, sometimes, radiation therapy or cryotherapy (freezing). Surgery is usually avoided, to prevent formation of another keloid.

Keratotomy, radial. A surgical procedure performed on the cornea (in the eye), to correct nearsightedness. *See also* Eye disorders, nearsightedness; Photorefractive keratectomy.

Kidneys. A pair of organs located behind the upper abdomen, just under the ribs. The kidneys' main function is to filter wastes from circulating blood, and eliminate this waste in urine. The urine flows through the ureter attached to each kidney, and is stored in the urinary bladder until it passes from the body. A person who loses a kidney due to injury or disease can manage with only one kidney, which then performs for both.

People with severe kidney disease who lose kidney function may be treated with a process called hemodialysis. The functions of the kidneys are performed by a machine that washes the blood and gets rid of wastes. Alternatively, a person who has lost kidney function may receive a kidney transplant, from a close relative or from another compatible donor. The new kidney takes on the functions of the person's defective kidneys.

Kissing disease. *See* Mononucleosis.

L

Labia. The outer lips of the vagina. *See also* Reproductive system, female.

Lactation. Flow of breast milk after the birth of a baby.

Lactose intolerance. A chronic inability to digest lactose, a sugar contained in milk. Lactose intolerance may cause diarrhea and difficulty in gaining weight in children, and such symptoms as bloating, gas, nausea, diarrhea, and abdominal cramps in adolescents and adults. Treatment consists of a lactose-free diet, avoidance of milk and milk products, or use of modified milk products. Over-the-counter products (Lactaid, Dairy

Ease, and others) are available that supply the natural enzyme to help in the digestion of lactose.

Laminaria. Specially prepared seaweed that is inserted in the cervix during early pregnancy in preparation for a second trimester abortion. The seaweed softens the cervix, making it easier to perform a vacuum extraction procedure.

Laparoscopy. A diagnostic procedure in which a thin, flexible, lighted tube is inserted through an incision into the lower abdomen. During the procedure the doctor looks for problems in the pelvic area that may affect the fallopian tubes, ovaries, or uterus. In some cases, corrective surgery may be done at the same time.

Laser. A device that produces a thin, intense beam of light that may be used as a cutting tool in some surgical procedures and in other medical treatments.

Lead poisoning. A chronic condition that can flare up from time to time into acute episodes. Lead poisoning occurs when the blood level of lead, normally present in blood in tiny (trace) amounts, is elevated. Lead poisoning causes symptoms such as headache, lack of appetite, a metallic taste, weakness, abdominal pain, vomiting, and constipation.

Lead poisoning can develop from eating lead-contaminated food (food or liquid stored in lead-glazed containers may become contaminated), or inhaling fumes of leaded gasoline or lead-contaminated dust over a period of time.

Children with significant levels of lead poisoning usually have severe symptoms that start suddenly and include violent vomiting spells. Small children who live in old buildings may develop lead poisoning from licking or chewing flakes of the old paint on the walls or on furniture (paint containing lead is no longer in use). Licking leaded pencil tips may also lead to elevated lead levels in blood.

Treatment consists of chelating agents that combine with the lead, which is then excreted in urine. Patients receiving chelating therapy may need to be hospitalized so the treatment can be monitored.

Learning disabled. A term that describes a person who has difficulty in understanding information taught in school or another educational facility. Learning disability may be due to an inherited or an acquired, mental or physical disorder or brain injury.

Many learning disabilities such as poor reading or writing skills can be overcome with the help of educational specialists, psychological counseling, physical therapy, practice, perseverance, and patience.

Lesbian. A female who is sexually attracted to other females.

Leukemia. A cancerous disorder of the blood that causes it to produce abnormal white blood cells. In past times, leukemia was almost always fatal. Today various types of leukemia can be cured by powerful new medications and other treatment methods.

Leukocyte. *See* White blood cell.

Leukocytosis. The presence of an excessive number of white blood cells in the blood. Extra numbers of white blood cells are produced when the body is fighting off an infection, and in certain blood diseases.

Leukopenia. The presence of fewer than the normal number of white blood cells in the blood. This condition may be found in a person who has a viral infection. Fewer white blood cells are produced in the bone marrow at such a time; consequently there is a smaller supply of white blood cells in the bloodstream.

Lice, head. Tiny organisms that cling to the hair and get nourishment by sucking blood from the host's skin. Lice bites cause severe itching. The eggs of lice (nits) are white, and are large enough to be visible. Head lice spread easily when people are in close contact, as in a school or camp.

A student's head lice should be reported promptly to the teacher and the school health office. Medicated shampoos and other procedures are used to kill the lice; the nits are removed with a special comb. Hats and other clothing in contact with the lice should be washed in very hot water and dried in a hot dryer. Clothes that are not washable should be discarded.

Lice, pubic. Tiny organisms called *P. pubis*, or crabs. The lice infest the pubic hair area and easily spread to other persons during close physical contact or contact with towels, sheets, or clothing. People infested with pubic lice usually complain of intense itching.

Treatment includes washing the pubic area with Elimite or Eurax shampoo. All clothing and bedding must be thoroughly cleansed in order to get rid of the resident lice.

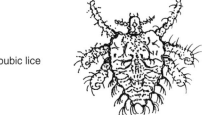

pubic lice

Ligament. Tough fibrous tissue that connects and supports bones and some other tissues.

Ligament, torn. An injury to a ligament, usually suffered during sports activity or an accident. Treatment for a mild to moderate tear includes Rest, Ice, Compression, and

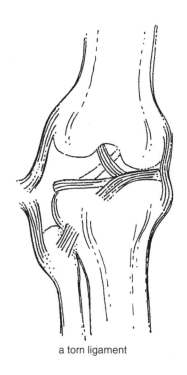
a torn ligament

Elevation (RICE) of the affected part. A severe tear may require surgery. *See also* RICE.

Lipectomy. *See* Liposuction.

Liposuction (suction lipectomy). A surgical procedure to suction out excess body fat through a small incision. This procedure can be used only for a healthy person with a specific fat problem—for example, large fat deposits in the thighs. This procedure should never be used in place of a weight loss program or appropriate diet and exercise.

Little League elbow. Painful elbow joint. Little League elbow often occurs when teens place excessive stress on their arms—as in too much throwing, or throwing special pitches such as curves and sliders—before their elbows are mature enough to handle such strenuous activities.

Liver. An essential organ, situated on the right side of the abdominal cavity. The liver stores digested food it receives from the small intestine and releases it, along with vitamins and other essential substances, to the body as needed.

The liver detoxifies wastes and poisonous materials in the body by removing them from the blood, and by destroying worn-out blood cells and hormones the body cannot use. Among many additional functions, the liver stores glycogen, which it converts to sugar and releases into the bloodstream when the blood sugar level is too low. Finally, the liver makes bile, which is essential for digestion. *See also* Digestive system.

Locking knee. A locking knee is caused by a piece of meniscus (the knee's shock absorber) that breaks off and becomes wedged in the knee joint. The knee freezes in the extended or bent position and cannot be moved. A knee that locks repeatedly may require surgery (meniscectomy) to restore normal knee function.

Lockjaw. *See* Tetanus.

Low body weight. *See* Underweight.

Low-risk behavior. Activities not likely to harm those involved.

Low self-esteem. Feelings of being "unworthy," or "no good." A person who has such feelings may be depressed. *See also* Depression.

LSD (Lysergic acid diethylamide). A substance used by some people to achieve a high, or various other altered mental states. Use of LSD is very risky. A person under the influence of LSD may have a "bad trip" and perform dangerous activities, such as jumping from a high place, in the belief that he or she can't be hurt. Other effects of LSD include flashbacks and hallucinations (misguided perceptions that lead to dangerously poor judgment), and these may recur for many months, sometimes even years. *See* Appendix C, Hallucinogens.

Lubricant. A substance used to reduce friction. Lubricants are often used during sexual activity. They include saliva or K-Y jelly, a water-based substance available in drugstores. *Note: Do not use petroleum jelly (Vaseline) with a condom; it will damage the condom and make it ineffective.*

Lues. Syphilis.

Lumbar puncture (LP). A diagnostic procedure used to determine whether infection, disease, or another abnormality is present in the spinal tract or central nervous system. A sterile needle is inserted through the back and into the spinal canal. A sample of spinal fluid is withdrawn and examined. A lumbar puncture is also performed when spinal anesthesia is given during surgery or childbirth.

Lupus erythematosus (LE) (cutaneous, chronic discoid). A disorder marked by reddish skin lesions that affect the face, the ears, and sometimes the upper trunk. The cause is unknown. Treatment consists of avoiding sunlight, using sunscreen when exposure is unavoidable, and applying cortisone ointment or cream. This condition may progress to a more serious form of lupus that affects many other body organs. *See* Systemic lupus erythematosus.

Luteinizing hormone (LH). A hormone produced in the brain that stimulates the monthly release of the egg from the ovary. *See also* Menstrual cycle.

Lyme disease. An infection caused by the bite of a tick carrying the infectious bacterium, the spirochete, *Borrelia* burgdorferi. When the tick bites a person or domestic animal and feeds on the blood, the infectious organisms can enter the bloodstream. There are many different kinds of ticks, but the deer tick (which feeds on deer) is the most common carrier of the infectious bacterium.

Symptoms of Lyme disease vary, and may mimic other illnesses. Early symptoms include a red rash at the site of the bite, sore

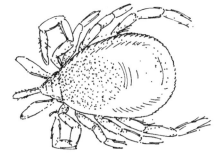

a deer tick

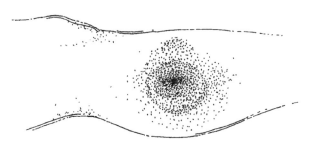

the characteristic bull's-eye rash of Lyme disease

throat, fever, fatigue, sleeping problems, a stiff neck, pain in joints and muscles, dizziness, and swollen glands. Weeks or even months later, there may be stiffness in the large joints, arthritis, and still other symptoms. A blood test may determine the diagnosis of Lyme disease, but it is not always reliable.

Treatment consists of antibiotics (amoxicillin, doxycycline), for fourteen to twenty-one days. If symptoms persist, intravenous antibiotics such as ceftriaxone (Rocephin) cefotaxime (Claforan), or penicillin may be given, usually for fourteen to twenty-one days. Early treatment is important to avoid complications.

To prevent Lyme disease, avoid fields and wooded areas where ticks live. Wear long pants, high socks, and other clothing to cover your arms and legs so that ticks cannot reach the skin, bite and attach themselves, and feed on blood.

An insect repellent with 20 to 30 percent of the chemical DEET may be applied to clothing, but should be kept away from the skin.

After an outing where ticks and deer are common, check clothing and the body for ticks. If any ticks are found, carefully brush them off, if possible. If the tick is attached to the skin, use fine tweezers to gently grab the tick near its mouthparts and pull it slowly out of the skin. Don't squeeze the tick. Save the tick in a small container, add a few drops of alcohol, and write down the date and the location of the bite. It will help the doctor or clinic to identify the insect, and make the correct diagnosis.

Lymphadenopathy. Enlargement of the lymph glands. This condition is usually found when an infection is present in a nearby part of the body, or in the presence of various other diseases.

Lymph glands. Glands that filter bacteria and viruses from the bloodstream. Lymph glands also produce antibodies and lymphocytes. These agents help the body to kill harmful organisms. *See also* Immune system.

Lymph node. A tissue sac that contains lymph glands.

Lymphatic system. A system composed of lymph glands, nodes, and the spleen. The lymphatic system links lymph glands, which contain lymphocytes produced in the bone marrow and in the thymus, a gland situated in the front of the neck.

Lymphocytes are white blood cells that prevent infection in several ways. They can recognize infectious organisms and other foreign invading substances, and fight them off before they can damage the body.

The lymph nodes also serve to catch foreign organisms, so that they can't spread infection. During such battles, the lymph glands in certain body areas become swollen, indicating that they are fighting an infection.

The spleen is a very large lymph gland in the back of the upper abdomen. It produces blood cells in the embryo, and later acts as a disposal station for worn-out red blood cells. *See illustration* The Human Body.

Lymphocyte. A cell that functions as one of the body's infection fighters. Lymphocytes consist of two types of cells: B cells and T cells. If these cells are in short supply, the body's defenses against infection and other harmful conditions are weakened, causing immunodeficiency (impaired immune system). *See also* Immune system; Lymphatic system.

Lymphoma. A type of cancer that causes a tumor in lymph tissues. There are two main types of lymphoma: Hodgkin's disease, and non-Hodgkin's lymphoma. Initial symptoms inlcude one or more swollen glands in the neck, armpit, or groin, and feelings of illness. The disease is diagnosed by examining (or removing) the swollen gland, and by blood tests. Treatment depends on the type of lymphoma diagnosed, and may consist of anticancer drugs, radiation therapy, and, sometimes, a bone marrow transplant to replace cells destroyed by the other treatment processes. Another procedure, plasmapheresis, may also be used. It involves removal of blood from the patient's vein, then removing unwanted blood components, and reinjecting the blood at a later time. *See also* Hodgkin's disease.

M

Magnetic resonance imaging (MRI). A diagnostic process that uses a scanning device, a magnetic field, and radio waves to penetrate bone tissue. The MRI allows examination of soft tissue beneath the bone

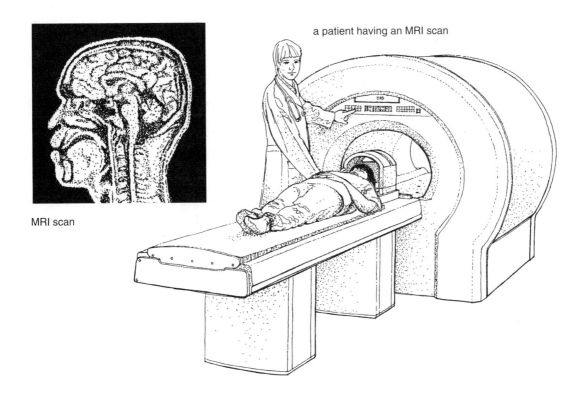

MRI scan

a patient having an MRI scan

and detection of abnormal conditions such as swelling or a tumor of the brain or spinal cord, and abnormalities in other body areas.

Malaise. General feeling of being ill, weak, or fatigued.

Malaria. A chronic infection caused by a parasite, and transmitted to humans bitten by infected *Anopheles* mosquitoes. Most malaria infections occur in tropical countries, but infected people may enter or return to the United States and bring in the disease. Malaria may also be transmitted through a blood transfusion from an infected donor, or through sharing of drug equipment, such as syringes or needles, by infected drug addicts. Once the parasite gets into the bloodstream, it causes chills, fever, sweating, anemia, and other symptoms.

The choice of an effective drug depends on which of four species of the parasite caused the illness. Incomplete treatment, or resistance to the drugs used, may lead to recurrent bouts of illness.

Anyone traveling to an area where malaria is present should take these preventive measures: use insect repellent and mosquito netting over the bed, and take prescribed antimalarial drugs.

Malignant. Describes a dangerous condition, such as a cancer.

Malignant melanoma. A rapidly invasive type of skin cancer that develops from the pigmented portion of the skin, and sometimes from a mole that suddenly starts to grow and spread. This type of lesion may be present at birth, rarely during adolescence, and usually becomes noticeable only in middle age or even later.

A malignant melanoma may be difficult to recognize, may appear anywhere on the body in different colors, or as a small, irregular bump. If you have a skin lesion—for example, a mole that changes color or size, starts to bleed, or itches—visit a dermatologist. This specialist diagnoses the lesion and provides appropriate treatment. Do not delay this examination. It may be fatal if not treated. Treatment, if needed, consists of surgical removal of the lesion and the surrounding areas. Avoidance of excessive exposure to sun and use of a good sunscreen are protective measures. *See also* Mole.

Malocclusion. A condition in which the upper teeth don't properly meet the lower teeth when chewing or when the mouth is closed.

Mammogram. An X ray of the breast tissues to detect and diagnose abnormal conditions.

Mammoplasty. Surgery to change the shape, or increase or decrease the size of a woman's breasts.

Mandatory. Required. Government regulations require (mandate) that patients diagnosed with an infectious disease such as gonorrhea, syphilis, AIDS, or tuberculosis be reported to state public health authorities. These diseases are highly contagious and can spread quickly through the population. Public health services record reported cases and prescribe public health measures to prevent further spread.

Mania. A psychological disorder. Symptoms include uncontrollable, wild behavior, sometimes with aggression and violence, extravagant spending, promiscuous sex, and rapid speech. A manic person may feel a sudden need to do or to have something that is out of his or her reach physically or economically. There are many possible causes for this abnormal mental state, including inherited mental disorder, acquired mental disorder due to biochemical disturbances, or substance abuse. Psychiatric treatment and medications are used to control manic behavior.

Manic depression. *See* Bipolar disorder.

MAP. *See* Morning-after pill.

Marijuana. A substance derived from the plant *Cannabis sativa*. Some people smoke marijuana to get high. Marijuana use is dangerous because it

- Is habit-forming
- Affects the user's mind, changing normal reactions to abnormal ones
- Alters a person's normal sense of time
- May cause the user to see things and hear voices that aren't there

Long-term use of marijuana is likely to cause loss of memory and a lack of interest in friends, family, and any activities other than smoking marijuana.

Massage. A treatment used for a variety of ailments, primarily sore muscles, spasms, or tension in various parts of the body. A massage involves rubbing, kneading, stretching, or using friction to manipulate a body part for a period of time. A person with back pain, for example, may receive a back massage; another person with leg or thigh muscle spasms may be treated with a massage in those areas.

There are many different massage techniques, including Swedish massage, Shiatsu, and others.

Masturbation. Manipulation of one's genitals to reach orgasm (sexual climax).

Masturbation, mutual. Stimulation of each other's genitals by two or more sexual partners to reach orgasm (sexual climax).

Mature onset of diabetes in the young (MODY). A rare mild form of diabetes mellitus in a child, teenager, or young adult. *See also* Diabetes mellitus.

Maximal breathing capacity (MBC). The total amount of air a person can breathe in one minute; also called maximal voluntary ventilation.

Maximal voluntary ventilation (MVV). *See* Maximal breathing capacity (MBC).

Measles (rubeola). A contagious disease that usually occurs during childhood or early adolescence.

Cause: A paramyxovirus.

Transmission: By way of airborne droplets from an infected person's nose or mouth.

Symptoms: Fever and headache, cold-like feelings, an itchy red rash that spreads from the face to the arms and body and appears as Koplik spots inside the mouth. Koplik spots occur only with measles and so confirm the diagnosis. Symptoms usually disappear after about five days.

Treatment: No specific treatment. The doctor usually prescribes bed rest, lotions for the itchy rash, and isolation of the patient to prevent spread of the infection. A vaccine, given to infants and young children, prevents measles. *See also* Immunization.

Measles, German (rubella). A contagious disease usually contracted during childhood or early adolescence.

Cause: An RNA virus.

Transmission: Through physical closeness to an infected child or through airborne droplets from an infected child's nose or mouth.

Symptoms: A general feeling of illness (malaise), coughing, swelling of the glands in the neck and behind the ears, and a rash inside the mouth and over the body. Symptoms usually last three to five days.

Treatment: No specific treatment except rest. A vaccine given to infants and young children prevents the disease. *See also* Immunization.

Complications: A woman who develops German measles during pregnancy may transmit the disease to her baby, who may be born with serious abnormalities.

Meatus. An opening in the body—for example, the urinary meatus, the opening of the urinary tube located at the tip of the penis or above the vagina. The urinary meatus discharges urine from the body.

Melanoma. *See* Malignant melanoma.

Membrane. A thin elastic sheet of tissue that covers some organs and lines the inner surface of others.

Menarche. The start of menstruation. Most girls start to menstruate between ages twelve and fourteen, although some have their first period as early as age ten, or as late as fourteen or older. A girl who has not had any periods by age fifteen or sixteen should have a

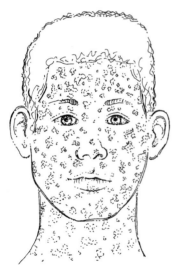

the characteristic measles rash

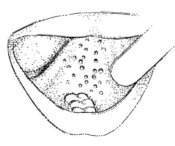

Koplik spots inside the mouth

checkup to make sure no medical problems are present. *See also* Menstruation.

Meningitis. Inflammation of the membranes that cover the brain and spinal cord.

Cause: A variety of viral and bacterial organisms. The germs that cause meningitis may travel to the bloodstream and set up a life-threatening, body-wide infection. Meningitis can spread quickly among groups of young people living in close contact, such as in school, at camp, or in military barracks.

Symptoms: May start with a sore throat, followed by fever, severe headache, stiff neck, and vomiting. Viral meningitis usually resolves without specific treatment. Bacterial meningitis, if not promptly and effectively treated, quickly worsens. The patient may feel drowsy, become unconscious, or have seizures (convulsions). Death may occur in one to several days.

Treatment of bacterial meningitis: Depends on the causative organisms found in spinal fluid obtained by lumbar puncture, and in blood tests. *See* Lumbar puncture. Powerful antibiotics given immediately can save the patient's life.

Meniscus. Cartilage shaped like a half-moon, located between the thighbone (femur) and the shinbone (tibia). A meniscus cushions various parts of the knee by acting like a shock absorber.

Menstrual cramps (dysmenorrhea). *See* Cramps, menstrual.

Menstrual cycle. The monthly occurrence of certain events in a woman's body that allow her to become pregnant and bear children. This is how the menstrual cycle works:

1. During the first few days of the 28- to 30-day menstrual cycle (starting with day 1 of a woman's period), a portion of the thick lining of the uterus is discarded.

2. As the cycle progresses (days 5 to 15),

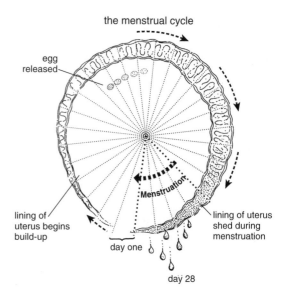

the menstrual cycle
egg released
lining of uterus begins build-up
Menstruation
lining of uterus shed during menstruation
day one
day 28

several hormones act to rebuild the uterine lining, in preparation for a possible pregnancy. The rich new lining will enable the uterus to nourish a fertilized egg as it becomes attached to the wall of the uterus.

3. At about mid-cycle (day 12 to 16), an egg is discharged from one of the ovaries. It passes through a fallopian tube and into the uterus.

4. If a woman has sex during this time, her partner's sperm may combine with the traveling egg and fertilize it.

5a. When the fertilized egg reaches the uterus, it may attach to the newly formed lin-

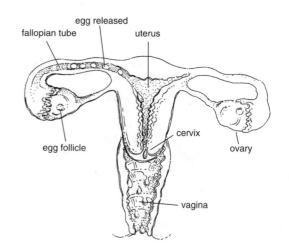

egg released
fallopian tube
uterus
egg follicle
cervix
ovary
vagina

ing, and a pregnancy can develop. If that happens, the woman will have no periods until after her baby is born.

5b. If the egg is not fertilized, the excess uterine lining is no longer needed. It separates from the wall of the uterus, causing the start of the period (usually during days 27 to 30 of the menstrual cycle). During menstruation, the unfertilized egg, the excess lining, and blood are discharged from the vagina.

6. The uterine lining returns to its previous thin, nonpregnant state, and the menstrual cycle starts over again.

This process is repeated every month during a woman's childbearing years, which may last from age eleven or twelve to age forty-five or longer. Once a woman reaches her late forties or fifties, her periods become less frequent and eventually stop.

Menstruation. The monthly discharge from the vagina of blood and uterine tissues, along with an unfertilized egg. This is a normal event that indicates the start of a new menstrual cycle. Menstruation starts in most girls at about ages twelve to fourteen. *See also* Menarche; Menstrual cycle.

Although girls start to menstruate at varying ages, a girl who has not had a period by age fifteen to sixteen needs a checkup, to see if a health problem is preventing the onset of her periods.

Some girls and women complain of discomfort during the days immediately before or during the period. This is a normal occurrence, caused by contraction of the uterine muscles as they squeeze out the excess uterine lining. Various measures can relieve menstrual discomfort. *See also* Cramps, menstrual.

Mental disease, disorder. A disorder of the mind. An otherwise healthy person who cannot cope with, or reacts abnormally to, the usual demands of daily life is suffering from a mental disease or disorder.

Many factors may produce a mental dis-order: a person who has great difficulty coping with stress, becomes deeply depressed, or suffers from great anxiety or mood swings may have, or may develop, a mental disorder. A mentally ill person is often unable to study, to work, to have a normal social life, and, instead, withdraws from normal contact with family members and friends.

Many mental disorders are due to biochemical processes in the brain that cause changes in thinking, behavior, and in emotional reactions. Mental disorders can be effectively treated with medication, psychotherapy, and combinations of these and other techniques. A psychiatrist usually diagnoses and treats serious mental disorders. Other mental health professionals (psychologists, psychiatric social workers) also treat mental disorders. *See also* Anxiety; Compulsion; Depression; Mania; Neurosis; Paranoia; Panic Attack; Personality disorder; Psychosis; Psychosomatic illness; Psychopath; Psychotherapy; Schizophrenia.

Mental health. A state of mind that allows a person to deal effectively with the demands of daily life. *See also* Mental disease, disorder.

Metabolism. The physical and chemical changes that must take place in all body tissues to keep them well nourished and functioning normally. Metabolism involves many complex processes that allow the body to convert food, water, and oxygen into living tissues, energy, and waste products.

Metastasis. The spread of abnormal cells from one part of the body to another. Cancer cells may travel from one body part to other areas, and thereby spread the disease. *See also* Cancer.

Middle ear infection. *See* Otitis media.

Migraine. A severe, sharp or throbbing headache that usually appears on the same side of the head. In some people migraine headache is caused by tension and stress. In others the cause is the intermittent contraction and subsequent relaxation of blood vessels in the brain. In some women, migraines appear most often before or during a period, indicating a hormonal cause. Other possible triggers include: lack of or too much sleep, low blood sugar, caffeine, wine, cheese, nuts, and birth control pills.

During a migraine headache a person may experience nausea, vomiting, and intense sensitivity to light and noise. Some people develop light sensitivity even before the migraine starts, giving them advance warning (aura, prodromal symptoms). Some people have migraine headaches only occasionally; others have them often.

Treatment includes over-the-counter pain relievers such as Tylenol, relaxation techniques, and avoidance of stress and other triggers. If these measures don't help, a doctor can prescribe medication to relieve head pain. Newer prescription medications that are taken daily reduce the frequency of migraine headaches and, in many cases, prevent them.

Minerals. Elements found in food that are essential for body functions. The body needs different minerals for various purposes, including good health and normal, efficient body functioning. A poorly balanced diet may lead to mineral deficiencies. *See also* Food groups; Nutition; Vitamins.

Minerals for your body's good health

Mineral	Benefit	Food Sources
Calcium	helps bone and teeth formation, blood clotting, nerve and muscle function	green leafy vegetables, tofu, low-fat dairy foods, eggs, beans, nuts
Chromium	helps the body use carbohydrates	lean meat, seafood, vegetables, fruits, seafood
Copper	helps the body use iron, protects bones	shellfish, beans, nuts, grapes, dried fruit, mushrooms
Fluorine	aids in bone and teeth formation	fluoridated water, fish, soybeans
Iodine	needed by the thyroid gland	iodized salt, saltwater fish, shellfish
Iron	promotes health of red blood cells, carries oxygen to body cells	lean meat, liver, fish, egg yolks, nuts, beans, some vegetables, raisins
Magnesium	aids nerve and muscle function, helps the body use energy	nuts, soybeans, low-fat dairy foods, green vegetables
Manganese	protects bones, helps the body use carbohydrates	green vegetables, nuts, beans, rice, oats
Phosphorus	helps in bone and teeth formation, needed for energy	lean meat, fish, poultry, beans, low-fat dairy foods
Potassium	helps in nerve and muscle function	green leafy vegetables, bananas, cantaloupe, low-fat milk, fish, nuts, potatoes
Selenium	guards body cells and tissues	lean meat, seafood, low-fat milk, whole-grain cereals
Sodium	aids nerve and muscle function, needed for body fluid balance	salt, bread, cereals, low-fat dairy foods
Zinc	needed for growth, energy	lean meat, seafood, poultry, nuts, beans, whole-grain cereals

Minnesota multiphasic personality inventory (MMPI). A psychological test used to evaluate personality and to diagnose mental illnesses such as depression or schizophrenia.

Minor, emancipated. An adolescent under age eighteen who lives independently, is self-supporting, and manages his or her own financial affairs, or is a parent.

Minor, mature. An adolescent age fifteen or older who is considered able to give informed consent to a recommended medical procedure. A mature minor can understand the reasons given by a health professional for the need to perform certain procedures, as well as their likely risks and benefits.

Miscarriage. Expulsion of an embryo (a pregnancy of three months or less) from the uterus. Most miscarriages occur during the early weeks of a pregnancy. Causes for miscarriage, also called "spontaneous abortion," are many. They include defects in a woman's reproductive system, hormonal imbalance, illness, infection, drug use, or a problem with the embryo.

After a miscarriage, a woman needs a prompt medical examination to make sure all embryo tissues were discharged from the uterus. If this is not done, infection and other problems may follow. Few women have more than one miscarriage. A woman who has more than one, however, may want to consult a fertility specialist. This medical expert will search for the cause and provide help in preventing future miscarriages.

Mitral valve prolapse (MVP). A common, usually harmless abnormality of the mitral valve (a flap of tissue located in the left side of the heart), which controls the flow of blood from the upper to the lower heart chamber. The mitral valve prevents the return of blood from the lower into the upper chamber. When the mitral valve does not close completely—that is, when it prolapses—some blood leakage may occur between the chambers.

A doctor listening to the heart of a person with MVP hears a characteristic murmur and a clicking sound. Tests may be needed to rule out other heart abnormalities. Some people have no symptoms: the MVP murmur is found during a routine physical examination. Others complain of chest pain while exercising; still others may feel pain or palpitation even while at rest.

These special precautions are recommended:
- A person who has MVP must take antibiotics before undergoing dental or other procedures that involve the opening of body tissues. This will prevent infection of the heart and surrounding tissues.
- Any person with or without MVP who has chest pain should have a medical examination, to rule out other heart problems that may require treatment.

Mole. A small or larger mass of tissue composed of skin cells that produce pigment, giving the mole its dark color. A mole is harmless unless it changes in size or shape, bleeds, or itches. When that happens, prompt examination by a dermatologist is needed, to make sure it is not a skin cancer (melanoma). If it is, it must be treated quickly, usually by surgery.

Molluscum contagiosum. A skin condition usually spread by direct physical or sexual contact.
Cause: A DNA pox virus.
Symptoms: Raised lesions or groups of lesions on the genitals and pubic area, or sometimes on the legs, trunk, or face. The nodules usually do not itch, but may produce a white discharge.
Treatment: Removal of the nodules by applying medication or by surgery.
Complications: Secondary infection of the affected areas due to scratching.

Special precautions: No sex until lesions are cleared up.

Moniliasis. *See* Candidiasis.

Monoamine oxidase inhibitor (MAOI). A drug used in the treatment of severely depressed people. *See also* Appendix B: Medications.

Monogamous. Having a sexual relationship with only one person.

Mononucleosis (infectious mononucleosis, kissing disease). A contagious viral infection most often seen in teenagers and young adults.

Cause: Epstein-Barr virus (EBV).

Transmission: Mainly by way of saliva. Infectious mononucleosis is known as the "kissing disease" because it is transmitted mainly through contact with the saliva of an infected person, possibly through kissing. It is not transmitted very easily, however. Poor hygiene and crowded living conditions are often responsible for spreading the infection.

Symptoms: Fever, headache, sore throat, enlarged lymph glands. Some people develop a red rash on the trunk and an enlarged liver and spleen.

Treatment: No specific treatment. Bed rest is needed while the person runs a fever and feels ill. Saline gargles for sore throat and medication such as Tylenol can relieve headache and other flulike symptoms.

Special precautions: No close contact with others while the illness lasts and for several weeks to months thereafter.

Monophasic birth control pills. *See* Birth control pill.

Moods. States of mind. Moods can change from happy to sad, and in other ways, often depending on events in a person's life. Pleasant events may lead to good moods—for ex-

ample, when a new boyfriend or girlfriend appears, when your team wins in a soccer game, or when you are doing well in school. You may become sad when a friend no longer wants to spend time with you or moves away, or when someone close to you is very ill or dies.

Angry feelings may arise during an argument with a friend, when someone you trust breaks a promise, or when parents say no to a request that is important to you.

Mood danger signals: A mood becomes a problem if it is too strong a response to the event that provoked it, or if it can't be controlled. For example, sadness that continues long after an event, or anger that is out of proportion to what a situation warrants, can be serious obstacles to normal life. Continued sadness can become a full-time occupation, leaving no time for fun and causing you to hang out by yourself, to do poor work in school, to eat too little or too much, and to feel seriously depressed.

Similarly, constantly angry people cannot enjoy life. They get angry at friends, and avoid sports and social activities, because they are preoccupied with their anger. These moods can be so overwhelming that a person may become depressed or violent, or both. A deeply depressed person often feels worthless, believes there is no point in being alive, and may wish to die. If these feelings are strong enough, if they persist for some time, and if nothing is done about them, that person may try to commit suicide.

Monitor your moods: If you feel sad or angry more often than you feel good about the way things are going in your life, talk to someone: a counselor, someone in your school health clinic, a doctor, or a religious leader. Discussing your feelings with someone else may help. If these advisers think you need more extensive help, they can refer you to a mental health professional who will help you to understand and deal with these harmful feelings.

Morning-after pill (MAP), Postcoital contraceptive (PCC), "911 pill." A specifically timed dosage of birth control pills taken shortly after sexual intercourse. This pill prevents pregnancy in almost all cases if taken within seventy-two hours of unprotected sexual intercourse. It contains the hormones estrogen and progesterone, which prevent the release of the egg from the ovary and the implanting of the egg in the uterine lining. Ovral is the MAP most often prescribed. Two pills are taken first, and two more are taken exactly twelve hours later. Other birth control pills may be prescribed, with different dosages and timing. *See also* Birth control.

Morning sickness. Nausea and vomiting during the first three months of pregnancy. The cause of morning sickness is not exactly understood, but it is probably due to the many glandular changes that take place at the start of pregnancy. Although morning sickness is a normal part of pregnancy, it is important for the pregnant woman to eat and drink adequate amounts in order to stay well nourished and hydrated. Many pregnant women find they can best tolerate frequent small meals of fairly bland foods and liquids. If nausea and vomiting are extreme, medical help is needed to ensure that mother and baby receive adequate nourishment.

Mouth to Mouth resuscitation. *See* Appendix F: First Aid.

MRI. *See* Magnetic resonance imaging.

Mucous membrane. The lining of the nose, throat, lungs, intestinal and genitourinary tract. It consists of skin cells that secrete mucus, a whitish, moist, protective substance that aids in the transport of fluids and other substances produced in these organs.

Mucus. A thick liquid secreted by the cells of the mucous membranes. *See* Mucous membrane.

Multiple sclerosis (MS). A disorder of the nervous system. The cause is unknown. The disease affects more women than men, usually beginning in ages twenty to forty. The disease affects the protective covering of nerve tracts (myelin). Symptoms include numb or tingling sensations, then progress to weakness, unsteadiness, muscle spasms and others, depending on the severity of the disease. Some medications can relieve symptoms, and treatments that may prevent the progression of the disease are being studied. There is no cure at this time.

Mumps. A contagious viral disease that is usually contracted during childhood.
  Cause: A paramyxovirus.
  Transmission: Contact with droplets of infected saliva or with an infected person's mouth.
  Symptoms: Chills, fever, general malaise, headache, and swelling of the salivary glands below and in front of the ears. Severe swelling causes pain during chewing or swallowing, especially when eating acidic foods such as oranges or foods prepared with vinegar or lemon juice. Boys may develop a painful inflammation of the testicles.
  Treatment: No specific treatment. Symptoms are treated with bed rest for fever and malaise; Tylenol for headache, fever, and malaise; a soft, bland diet (no acidic foods) when glands are swollen; a soft support and an ice pack placed on the testicles provide relief if the scrotum is painful and swollen.
  Prevention: Infants immunized with mumps vaccine will not contract this infection. *See also* Immunization.

Muscle cramps. Pain most often in the

lower leg caused by muscle spasms. Cramps may develop after strenuous exercise, especially when it involves heavy perspiration and loss of water, which depletes blood potassium levels. Rest, massage of the painful area, moist heat, and careful stretching for a brief period will provide relief.

Muscle, pulled. A muscle injury in which muscle fibers are strained or torn. A pulled muscle may become tight and cause painful spasms. Loss or limitation of muscle function results, and lasts until healing is complete. Treatment includes Rest, Ice, Compression, and Elevation of the arm or leg (RICE). *See also* RICE.

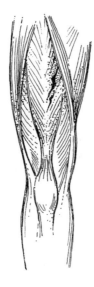

Muscular dystrophy. A muscle-wasting disease of unknown cause. This disease often occurs in families and may start during childhood. The muscles lose strength as the child grows older, making standing, walking, and other activities difficult or impossible.

There is no specific treatment for this disease. Depending on the extent of the muscle weakness, braces or a wheelchair can provide support and mobility. Physical therapy, massage, and exercise help to preserve muscle tone.

Mycobacterium avium intracellulare (MAI) infection. An infection similar to tuberculosis in the lung or another organ. MAI is an opportunistic infection; it seizes the opportunity to develop in a person with a defective immune system, as is the case with AIDS.

Myopathy. A muscle disease, abnormality.

Myopia. *See* Eye disorders.

N

Natural family planning. *See* Rhythm method.

Naturopathy. The use of nature to treat illness and preserve health. Treatments include sunbaths, a vegetarian diet, use of steam, and others.

Nausea. An uneasy, queasy, or sick sensation in the stomach, sometimes accompanied by vomiting. Nausea can be caused by viral or bacterial infections, various illnesses, some medications, alcohol, and stress.

Nearsightedness. *See* Eye disorders.

Necrosis. Death of body tissue. May result from infection or other causes.

Nervous, nervousness. A state of feeling anxious or agitated due to stress. A nervous person may have a dry mouth, sweaty palms, an increased heart rate with a sensation of fluttering or skipping a heartbeat (palpitation), stomach distress, headache, and other symptoms.

Feelings of nervousness may be due to the release of the body chemical adrenaline, which arms the body for a struggle or emergency. When the stressful incident is over, the body relaxes. With frequent or long-lasting stress, other symptoms—such as exhaustion or depression—may appear.

A teen who is frequently nervous needs to talk with a trusted friend, teacher, counselor, or physician to identify and overcome the nervousness.

Nervous system. A large group of interconnected structures that govern all body functions. The nervous system consists of the brain, spinal cord, and an immense network of nerves extending through the body.

The basic unit of this system is the one-celled neuron.

The nervous system controls all body actions by conducting impulses from the brain (the "master" of the nervous system) by way of nerve pathways to all parts of the body and back to the brain, making it possible to think, move, breathe, see, and carry out all the other functions essential to life.

Different types of nerve cells allow specific functions: Motor nerve cells make voluntary movement (of a limb, for example) possible. Sensory nerves bring messages to the brain from all parts of the body. The autonomic (involuntary) nervous system regulates involuntary body actions, such as breathing, the heartbeat, and intestinal functions. It consists of two parts: the sympathetic nervous system, made up of nerves that speed up body activities, and the parasympathetic nervous system, with nerves that slow them.

When a person is in danger, for example, the sympathetic nervous system automatically increases the heart rate, respirations, and secretions from various glands to allow coping with the emergency. Afterward, the parasympathetic nervous system goes into action to slow body activities back to normal.

Neurological. Refers to the nervous system.

Neurosis. An emotional disorder less severe than a psychosis. There are many possible causes of neuroses. They include excessive fears (phobias), anxiety, or the desire for perfection. Specific fears may be felt or expressed, for example, a fear of being shut in (claustrophobia); or at a great height (acrophobia); excessive concern about cleanliness, or about sex. These fears and anxieties can make ordinary daily life difficult or impossible.

Neuroses can be overcome with psychotherapy, counseling, and medications. *See also* Phobia; Psychosis.

Nevus. *See* Mole.

Night sweat. Drenching perspiration that occurs during sleep at night. Night sweat is one of the symptoms of tuberculosis.

Nipples, inverted. Nipples that point into the breast instead of outward. Some girls, as well as some boys, are born with this condition. It is no cause for concern unless the inverted position of the nipples interferes with functions such as nursing a baby. A breast shield can be used to overcome this problem.

Nipples that point outward, then invert to point inward, need to be examined by a physician. This change may signal an abnormal condition such as a tumor.

Nocturnal emission (wet dream). The involuntary release of semen (ejaculation) during sleep. This is a normal event experienced by most boys during early to middle adolescence (age thirteen to fifteen). It is not necessary to have a sexy dream for nocturnal emission to occur.

Nocturnal enuresis. *See* Enuresis.

Nongonococcal urethritis (NGU). Inflammation of the urethra (urinary tube) not caused by the gonococcus organism (the cause of gonorrhea). The cause of NGU may be a chlamydial or other infection. Symptoms include a burning sensation while urinating, increased urination, and a white or yellowish discharge from the penis. Some males have a slight tickling sensation in the penis. This disappears in a few days but the infection is still present and may be transmitted to a sex partner. *See also* Urethritis.

Non-Hodgkin's lymphoma. *See* Lymphoma.

Non-insulin-dependent diabetes mellitus (NIDDM, diabetes mellitus Type 2). *See* Diabetes mellitus.

Nonoxynol-9. A chemical agent that kills sperm. Nonoxynol-9 is commonly used along with contraceptive barrier devices such as the cervical cap, diaphragm, and condoms.

Nonspecific urethritis (NSU). *See* Urethritis.

Nonspecific vaginitis. *See* Vaginitis.

Normal. When used in health care, the term indicates that no illness, disease, infection, or other adverse condition is present.

Normal penis size. Many boys and men are concerned about the size and shape of their penis and wonder whether it is normal. In particular, some worry that their penis is too small.

Penis size—both width and length—is determined by hereditary and other factors. Studies have shown that during sexual arousal a small penis increases as much in size proportionately as a larger penis. The most important point is that penis size does not affect sexual performance or the ability to father a child.

Norplant. *See* Contraceptive.

Nosebleeds. An injury, cold, or infection can damage the membrane lining the nose and cause bleeding. *See* Appendix F: First Aid.

Nose job. *See* Rhinoplasty.

Nutrition. The provision of adequate, nourishing food that enables children to grow into healthy adults and allows adults to maintain strong, healthy bodies. *See also* Diet, Food groups, Food pyramid.

Nymphomania. An obsession with sex. The term is usually applied to women; satyriasis is used to describe the condition in men. A person with nymphomania or satyriasis tends to be preoccupied with sex and unable to concentrate on other important activities. These are emotional disorders that require treatment by a mental health professional.

Obesity. State of being overweight. Ideal weight is determined by height, age, sex, and body frame (small, medium, large). Excess weight may lead to serious medical problems.

If you think you are overweight, go to your school clinic or see your physician. These health professionals will tell you if you need to lose weight. They can help you choose an appropriate diet, and they will prescribe specific exercises. Once you start a healthy low-fat diet and begin regular exercise you will be on the way to achieving your weight reduction goal.

Obsessive-compulsive disorder. *See* Compulsion.

Oily hair and skin. A condition caused by unusually large amounts of oil secreted by oil glands located under the skin and near the hair follicles. Excessive oil may be produced in response to increased hormonal activity during the teen years, giving the face and scalp an oily appearance.

You can treat oily skin and hair by washing your face several times a day with soap, and shampooing your hair at least three times a week. Special soaps and shampoos for oily skin and hair can be found in a drugstore. A healthy diet is also helpful. If these measures don't produce results, your doctor can prescribe a stronger medicated soap and shampoo.

Oligomenorrhea. Infrequent and irregular periods. A woman with oligomenorrhea may menstruate occasionally, every few months, or even less frequently. Irregular or occasional periods are the result of a hormonal imbalance, very low weight, or other causes.

A medical checkup is essential to find the exact cause and determine the need for treatment. *See also* Menstruation.

Opportunistic infection (OI). An infection that occurs because the immune system is impaired, and unable to adequately defend the body against a virus or other organisms. A defective immune system allows the organisms to multiply, giving them the opportunity to start an infection. *See also* Immune system.

Oral contraceptive. A pill taken regularly to prevent pregnancy. The Pill usually contains the hormones estrogen and progesterone, or sometimes only progesterone. Oral contraceptives are generally safe and highly effective in protecting against pregnancy. The Pill is most effective when taken exactly as prescribed, under the supervision of a health professional. *See also* Birth control; Birth control pill; Contraceptive; Morning-after pill.

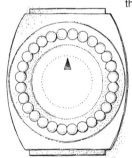

the Pill

a month's supply of oral contraceptive pills, arranged so that one pill is taken each day during the menstrual cycle

Oral sex. *See* Intercourse, sexual.

Orgasm. The climax of the sexual act.

Orthodontist. A dental specialist who straightens the teeth and corrects a poor bite, by applying dental braces or other devices.

Osgood-Schlatter disease. Inflammation of the main leg bone (tibia) near the knee joint. This disease occurs mainly in teenagers. Symptoms include a lump (swelling) and pain just below the knee. The pain is especially noticeable when climbing stairs.

If you have these symptoms, it is important to get a prompt medical examination to determine the cause of the pain. Several other conditions also produce leg or knee pain but require different treatment.

Osgood-Schlatter disease is treated with exercises to strengthen the large thigh (quadriceps) muscles, pain-relieving medication, and avoidance of pain-causing activities for some time.

Ostomy (colostomy, cystostomy, ileostomy). A surgically created opening in the bowel (colostomy), bladder (cystostomy), small intestine (ileostomy), or certain other sites. Such an opening may be needed when illness causes a blockage or damage in an organ, preventing normal function, or the normal discharge of stool or urine.

The ostomies described above allow a regular discharge of stool or urine, essential for normal body functioning. The discharge is collected in a bag attached to the body with adhesive or similar material and held in place by a belt. The bag is emptied as needed. In some cases, the surgeon creates an internal pouch by using body tissues. The discharge collects inside the pouch, and is removed through a tube (catheter) whenever necessary. In some cases, an ostomy may be reversed by surgery when it is no longer needed.

OTC, over-the-counter. A term used to indicate drugs such as pills, liquids, creams, ointments, lotions, and lozenges, available in drugstores without a doctor's prescription.

Otitis media. Inflammation of the middle ear, caused by irritation or infection. This painful condition often occurs in children after a cold or sore throat and sometimes after measles. Treatment consists of antibiotics and soothing ear drops.

Outercourse. Hugging, kissing, petting, and other means of expressing affection that do not involve vaginal or anal penetration (sexual intercourse).

Ova and parasites test (O&P). A laboratory test performed on a small quantity of stool, to look for the presence of worms, cysts, or eggs. *See also* Parasite infestation.

Ovarian cyst. A growth in the ovary that is filled with fluid or semisolid material. Cysts are generally benign but occasionally cancerous. They may be too small to be felt on examination or to cause symptoms. Cysts often appear and then disappear within a few months without treatment.

An ovarian cyst can grow rapidly to a very large size and cause pain, an enlarged abdomen, infection, and bleeding. Any of these symptoms require an immediate examination. Treatment depends on the size and type of cyst diagnosed.

Ovary. A female reproductive gland. A female has two ovaries, one on either side of the uterus. Each ovary contains many eggs. *See also* Ovulation; Menstrual cycle.

Over-the-counter. *See* OTC.

Overweight. *See* Obesity.

Ovulation. The release of an egg from the ovary. Ovulation usually occurs ten to fourteen days after the start of the menstrual cycle. From the ovary, the egg travels to the uterus over the course of about six days. If the egg meets a sperm and unites with it, the egg is fertilized. If the fertilized egg then reaches the uterus and settles safely in the uterine wall, a pregnancy results. *See also* Conception; Fertilization; Menstrual cycle; Menstruation.

Ovum. Egg. An egg is released from a woman's ovary each month and passes through the fallopian tube and into the uterus.

P

Pain. A sensation of discomfort or hurt somewhere in the body. Pain is a symptom; it indicates the presence of an injury, illness, infection, or, sometimes, a psychological condition in which stress or some other type of mental problem results in pain.

People react to pain in different ways, with some able to tolerate higher levels of pain than others. Mild, temporary pain or discomfort, such as a headache or a muscle ache, usually stops after a short time, or can be treated with rest and, sometimes, a mild pain reliever.

Moderate or severe pain is a warning sign, and requires medical investigation to find the cause. Severe abdominal pain, for example, may indicate an acute digestive upset, infection, appendicitis, or another type of illness. These conditions must be diagnosed and treated promptly, to avoid dangerous consequences.

Palpate. Feeling, or exerting gentle pressure wih the hands to feel the size, shape, and location of an organ, for example, the liver, to determine possible abnormalities (enlargement, unusual shape) during a physical examination. *See also* Physical examination.

Palpitation. A fluttering sensation in the chest, as if the heart is skipping a beat, or a throbbing heartbeat. Palpitations may occur when the heart beats faster or in an irregular fashion (arrhythmia). Palpitations sometimes occur after a strenuous run. They may be the result of stress, anxiety, excitement or nervousness, caffeine, some prescribed drugs, certain illicit drugs, infection, or, in rare cases, an abnormality of the heart. An occasional bout of palpitations does not necessarily mean something is wrong. A doctor should be consulted for prolonged or frequent bouts of palpitations. *See also* Arrhythmia.

Pancreas. An important gland located inside the abdomen, behind the stomach. The pancreas produces digestive juices and insulin, which is involved in the body's use of sugar and other carbohydrates. *See also* Digestive system.

Panic attack. A symptom that occurs from time to time in a person who suffers from anxiety. A panic attack usually occurs during a period of stress or great fear. Its symptoms are rapid respirations, a feeling of not getting enough air, a fast pulse, or chest pain that makes the person feel he or she is having a heart attack. Treatment includes counseling, medication, and a program to help the person to overcome fears and anxieties.

Pap smear (Papanicolaou smear). A test to detect certain infections and cancer of the cervix and uterus. An instrument is inserted in the cervical opening. Samples of cells are gently scraped from the lining of the cervix and from its outer surface, and examined in the laboratory to see if precancerous cells, cancerous cells, or an infection are present. Treatment can then be prescribed.

An annual Pap smear is needed for every sexually active woman. More frequent Pap smears may be needed for those who have had a sexually transmitted infection, or do not use condoms regularly with one or more male partners.

Paralysis. Inability to move, caused by a physical or psychological disorder or illness. A person's muscles may not function and therefore it is impossible for the person to move arms, legs, and other body parts, because the nerves needed for muscle movement are damaged, inactivated, or destroyed.

Some forms of paralysis are temporary, and are reversed once the underlying illness is treated. Other forms of paralysis may be permanent, for example, in a person who has suffered a spinal cord injury or illness in which nerves have been severed or destroyed.

Paranoid personality disorder. A mental disorder in which persons are extremely suspicious and believe that other people—real or imaginary—wish to harm them. *See also* Mental disease, disorder.

Paraphimosis. A congenital or, sometimes, acquired condition in which the foreskin has pulled back from the head of an uncircumcised penis and cannot be pulled forward again. Treatment consists of surgery.

Parasite. An organism that lives on, or inside another organism, from which it derives nourishment. A parasite, such as a worm or the tick that carries Lyme disease, often causes illness in the host. *See also* Parasite infestation.

Parasite infestation. An infection, usually of the intestinal tract, caused by bacteria or tiny organisms such as worms or their eggs. *See also* Parasite.

Parasite infections include amebiasis, giardiasis, and malaria, among others. Worm infestations include pinworms, hookworms, tapeworms, and other less common varieties.

Transmission: Parasite infestations are transmitted in various ways: by eating food contaminated by human or animal feces that contain the parasite, by drinking contaminated water, and by swimming or wading in infested ponds or streams. Certain tiny parasites may work their way into the skin of a person walking bare-

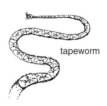
tapeworm

foot. Others may be transmitted through sexual contact. Some parasitic infections are rare in this country, but are common in other countries. They may be brought into the United States by immigrants or returning travelers. *See also* Malaria; Trichinosis.

Treatment: Depends on the parasite identification through laboratory tests. It may include antibiotics, other medications that kill specific parasites, and, occasionally, surgery.

Special precautions: Careful hand washing before handling food, after touching raw meat, and after using the toilet; boiling water not safe to drink or to use in preparing food, or using bottled water; wearing shoes to prevent parasite access into the feet; using certain public health measures to decontaminate infested waters; and taking preventive medications when traveling in countries where there is risk of parasite infestation.

Paronychia. An inflammation that develops as a result of infection around the base or side of a fingernail or a toenail. Swelling, redness, and pain are the symptoms. Treatment includes antibiotics or antifungals, depending on the infection. People who must keep their hands in water much of the time, or those who try to change the appearance of their cuticles are more likely to develop this problem. Anyone susceptible to this type of infection should wear rubber or plastic gloves when the hands are immersed in water, and refrain from damaging the cuticles.

Parotid (salivary) glands. The glands, one on each side of the face, in front of and below each ear. These glands are known as the salivary glands; they secrete saliva into the mouth.

Parotitis. An inflammation of the parotid (salivary) glands, situated in front of and be-low each ear. Parotitis may develop as a complication of mumps. *See also* Mumps; Parotid glands.

Patch test. A test to determine allergic reactions to various substances. A very small quantity of the test substance is placed on the skin. If an allergist observes a positive reaction after a few hours or a few days, the allergy is confirmed. *See also* Allergy; Skin tests.

Patellar tendinitis. Inflammation of the knee's major supporting tendon (the tough, fibrous band of tissue that connects muscle to bone). Treatment includes anti-inflammatory medications such as ibuprofen (Advil); Rest, Ice, Compression (Ace bandage), Elevation (RICE); and progressive exercises as prescribed by a physician. *See also* Tendinitis; RICE.

Pathogen. A microscopic organism such as a bacterium or a virus that can transmit a disease or infection from one person to another.

Pediculosis capitis. *See* Lice, head.

Pediculosis pubis. *See* Lice, pubic.

Peer pressure. Influence on each other by friends of the same age. The attitudes, likes, and dislikes of peers can often be a strong influence on young people. Being like their friends in behavior, hairstyles, clothing, choice of music, and other matters offers a feeling of being accepted by their peers.

Peer pressure affects teens' choices in ways that may be positive or negative. Teens who enjoy exercise, sports, and good nutrition exert *positive* peer pressure on their friends. Teens who use street drugs or experiment sexually at a very early age may exert *negative* peer pressure on friends who follow their example, hoping to keep their respect and friendship.

Pelvic examination. Medical examination

of a female's reproductive tract (vagina, cervix, uterus, and fallopian tubes) to determine if there are any problems. A pelvic examination may be part of a general physical checkup, or may be performed by a specialist in women's health (gynecologist). If the examiner is male, a female nurse or other health professional will usually remain in the room during the pelvic exam.

The examination is performed with the woman lying on her back on the examining table, covered with a sheet to preserve her privacy. The woman's legs are raised and placed in stirrups on either side of the table. This position allows the doctor to clearly see the genital area and to examine the internal reproductive organs. The examination is done in two parts:

1. A speculum (instrument to visualize the interior of the vagina) is placed into the vagina, to allow the examiner to inspect it and the cervix for any abnormalities. The woman can ask the doctor or health care provider to hold up a mirror, so she can see the inner parts of her body. *See illustration* The Human Body. Samples of vaginal and cervical fluid and cells are removed to be tested for infection, cancer, and other abnormalities. The speculum is then removed.

2. The doctor places two fingers into the vagina and gently presses upward, toward the abdomen. At the same time, the doctor's other hand gently presses on the woman's lower abdomen. This allows the physician to determine the size and shape of the internal organs and to detect any problems.

The woman may feel slight pressure but no pain during the examination, which lasts two to three minutes. Any severe discomfort should be reported to the examiner as it may indicate a problem.

Adult women should have pelvic examinations at regular intervals, to make sure the reproductive system is healthy and functioning normally. It may be helpful to make a list of questions or concerns about your body, birth control methods, or other topics to discuss after the examination. *See also* Pap smear.

Pelvic inflammatory disease (PID). A serious infectious disease of a female's pelvic organs (the uterus and fallopian tubes).
Cause: PID is almost always caused by one or more sexually transmitted diseases, which travel from the vagina into the uterus and fallopian tubes.
Transmission: Sex with a partner who is in-

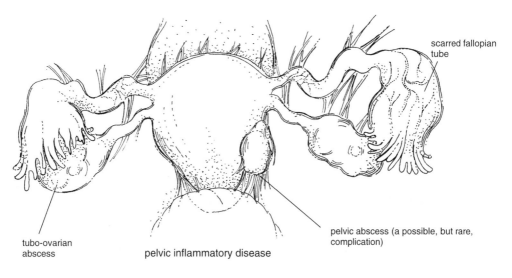

tubo-ovarian
abscess

pelvic inflammatory disease

scarred fallopian
tube

pelvic abscess (a possible, but rare, complication)

fected with one or more sexually transmitted diseases.

Symptoms: Severe pain, nausea, bleeding, and often a high fever.

Treatment: Strong antibiotics. Hospitalization may be necessary.

Complications: An abscess may develop if PID is not treated promptly. Other long-term complications include chronic pain, scar tissue in the fallopian tubes, sterility, and tubal pregnancy (pregnancy in one of the fallopian tubes).

Special precautions: No sex during acute phase of the illness.

Pelvis. The lower portion of the abdomen, which contains the pelvic bones, muscles, and other structures that support the organs located in the pelvic area. The pelvis contains the urinary bladder and the internal genital organs. *See illustration* The Human Body.

Penetration, sexual. The insertion of a penis, a finger, or a foreign object into a woman's vagina or a person's rectum.

Penis. The male sex organ, also called the phallus. *See also* Normal penis size.

Period. The phase in the menstrual cycle in which blood and tissues no longer needed are discarded by the uterus in the menstrual flow. *See also* Menstruation; Menstrual cycle.

Periodontist. A dentist who specializes in treating gum diseases.

Persistent generalized lymphadenopathy (PGL). A condition associated with HIV infection. Lymph glands in various parts of the body become swollen and remain in that state for weeks or months. *See also* AIDS.

Personality disorder. An emotional disorder that changes a person's behavior (personality) to the point that he or she is unable to deal with normal life situations and re-

quirements. Such a person may become suspicious of family members, friends, or other people, stay away from usual social contacts, and, in general, act strangely and not as before this problem appeared.

A psychiatric examination is needed to determine the cause, to be followed by treatment that may involve psychotherapy and medications.

Perspiration. Sweating. This normal function allows the body to cool off when hot. Perspiration is usually a healthy consequence of exercise, other exertion, or time spent in hot surroundings.

Teens often discover that their sweat glands become overactive when they are nervous or under stress, causing wet, clammy hands and heavy perspiration under the arms. This is normal. Perspiration tends to become more intense during adolescence, along with other physical changes. Self-conscious teens need to realize that they can learn to deal effectively with stress and anxiety. Any teen who is embarrassed by perspiration should remember that all people, not just teenagers, perspire at certain times.

To overcome the unpleasant effects of perspiration, take frequent baths or showers and use an underarm antiperspirant that absorbs moisture and prevents odor, or a deodorant that simply prevents odors. If necessary, girls can wear underarm shields under their clothing to absorb excessive moisture and prevent sweat stains.

Note: Any person who perspires heavily should drink fluids to make up for water lost by sweating. This is especially important in hot temperatures, where loss of body fluids may cause severe overheating, dehydration, and dangerous heatstroke. *See also* Dehydration.

Phallus. *See* Penis.

Phencyclidine (PCP). *See* Angel dust.

Phenylketonuria. A disease of newborn babies caused by the inability to utilize the amino acid, phenylalanine. Every baby is now tested for this disease at birth. If present, a diet low in phenylalanine prevents brain damage and other symptoms that will otherwise develop and cause mental retardation.

Phimosis. A condition in which the foreskin is so tight that it cannot be pulled away (retracted) from the head of the penis. A surgical procedure, circumcision, solves this problem.

Phobia. An excessive fear of certain people or situations; a psychological problem. Phobias appear in many different forms. Claustrophobia is a fear of closed-in spaces. A person who has claustrophobia cannot enter an elevator or other confined areas. Agoraphobia is a fear of open spaces. Afflicted people cannot leave home because of an overwhelming fear, which they cannot explain.

Phobias can cause people to restrict their daily activities. Certain mental health centers specialize in treating people with phobias and work to help them overcome their fears so they can live normal lives. *See also* Neurosis.

Photorefractive keratectomy (PRK). A new surgical procedure to correct mild to moderate nearsightedness. During the surgery, a laser is used to reshape the cornea, and so improve vision. The procedure is usually done on one eye, and three months later, on the other eye. It should not be used for severe nearsightedness. *See also* Eye disorders, nearsightedness.

Physical examination. A complete inspection of the body, its organs, and its various systems, including the skin, eyes, and ears; the nervous system; the cardiovascular system (heart, blood, and blood vessels); and the respiratory, musculoskeletal, genitouri-

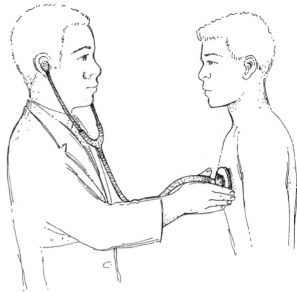

As part of the physical exam, the doctor uses a stethoscope to check the heart and lungs.

nary, and reproductive systems. By examining each body system, a health professional can determine a person's health status and detect conditions that need treatment or further study.

To start, the health professional takes an individual and family health history, checks vital signs (pulse, respirations, blood pressure), and measures height and weight. Hearing and eyesight and the respiratory system may be tested at this time.

A careful check for external evidence of any problems—for example, a lump, rash, or sign of an infection—is next. The doctor listens to the heart and lungs with a stethoscope to determine if the heart and lung sounds are normal. Nerve reflexes are tested by tapping the knees; and the arms, knees, and legs are checked for their ability to move freely.

Palpation of the abdomen follows. The doctor places both hands on various parts of the belly to feel internal organs such as the liver, to make sure no enlargement or growth is present.

A female may have a breast and a pelvic examination. *See* Pelvic examination; Breast self-examination.

A male may have a genital examination, which includes palpation of the testicles for lumps or tumors, and inspection of the penis for discharge or other problems. *See* Testicular self-examination.

Urine, blood, and other body fluid or tissue samples may be collected and sent to a laboratory for examination. A test may be done for tuberculosis. Other laboratory tests or procedures may be done if the examination shows they are needed. These may include a chest X ray and an electrocardiogram.

Once test results are available, they are evaluated along with the findings of the physical examination. The doctor then gives the examined person a complete report of his or her health status.

Note: The health care provider may not routinely check for sexually transmitted diseases (STDs). You may ask about tests for gonorrhea, syphilis, chlamydial infection, hepatitis, and other STDs.

Physical exercise. Use of the body to promote physical fitness; to improve muscle strength, breathing capacity, and circulation; and to increase a sense of well-being.

Piercing, of the ears, nose, and other body parts. While pierced earlobes have been popular for centuries, some people are now also having their noses, lips, navels, nipples, and other body areas pierced, to accommodate rings, studs, and other jewelry. Their motives vary. Some seek to make their bodies more attractive, others wish to indicate a rebellious attitude or to "make a statement" about themselves and their lifestyle, others are following a current fad.

Piercing of a body part generally begins with cleaning the skin and passing a specially designed sterile needle through the flesh. Immediately afterward, a sterile ring or other piece of jewelry of appropriate size and material (surgical quality stainless steel or 14-karat gold) is inserted.

Aftercare consists of cleaning the pierced area as well as the jewelry several times a day with antiseptic solution, then applying antibiotic ointment and moving (rotating) the jewelry through the hole to keep it open.

Caution: Have piercing performed only by a physician familiar with the procedure, or at a reputable piercing salon where appropriate equipment and sterilization techniques are used. If piercing is not properly done, infection with bacteria, viruses, or fungi may follow, with potentially serious consequences.

Pill, the. An oral contraceptive. *See* Contraceptive; Oral contraceptive.

Pill, morning-after. *See* Contraceptive; Morning-after pill.

Pimples. Small bumps on the skin, a common condition during the teen years. In adolescence, certain hormones become more active and stimulate oil glands located under the skin of the face, back, and chest to produce extra amounts of oil. Over time, white or black bumps may appear on the skin. If the oil becomes trapped under the skin, it may cause irritation. The body then reacts as it does to infection or inflammation: a hard, tender, red lump may develop.

To prevent or heal pimples, wash the face daily with soap and water to remove excess oil from the skin. If the skin breaks out in pimples in various places, a doctor or health clinic can provide a prescription that will clear up the pimples and prevent their recurrence. *See also* Acne; Appendix B, Acne medications.

Pinworm. *See* Parasite infestation.

Pituitary gland. An endocrine gland in the brain that secretes several essential hormones that regulate many aspects of growth, development, and body functions.

Placenta. A pancake-shaped tissue that develops in a pregnant woman's uterus to nourish the growing fetus through the pregnancy. *See also* Pregnancy.

Planned Parenthood Federation of America (PPFA). An organization devoted to research and counseling in family planning, birth control methods, treatment of sexually transmitted diseases and AIDS, and pregnancy prevention and termination. Clinics exist all over the country and are listed in local telephone directories.

Plantar wart. Overgrowth of skin on the sole of the foot, caused by a virus. A wart may press on the sole and cause pain while standing or walking. Over-the-counter wart-removal medications are available at drugstores. If these are unsuccessful, electrocautery is used to burn off the wart, or cryosurgery to freeze it, or a minor surgical procedure to remove it.

Whichever treatment is used, it is important to keep pressure off the wart. You can cut a circular hole in a piece of adhesive mole foam (soft padding available at the drugstore) and fit it around the wart. The foam prevents pressure, decreases pain, and aids in healing.

Warts may come back. If that happens, the treatment is repeated.

Plasmapheresis. *See* Hodgkin's disease.

Plastic and reconstructive surgery. A surgical procedure to repair damage to the body caused by illness or injury. It is also performed to improve the appearance of a misshapen or oversized body part. *See also* Liposuction; Mammoplasty; Rhinoplasty.

Platelet. A blood component that helps blood to clot. *See also* Blood.

PMS. *See* Premenstrual syndrome.

Pneumocystis carinii pneumonia (PCP). Inflammation of the lungs caused by the organism *Pneumocystis carinii*. Healthy people do not usually become ill when exposed to this organism. But a person with a defective immune system, as occurs with AIDS or cancer, may develop a severe PCP infection. *See also* Opportunistic infection.

Pneumoencephalogram (PEG). An X-ray examination of the brain, done after injecting air into the surrounding spaces to make the brain's structures more easily visible.

Pneumonia. Infection of the lungs, caused by harmful organisms that invade the respiratory passages. Symptoms include fever, chest pain, fluid buildup, shortness of breath, and a faster breathing rate. Treatment includes antibiotics and bed rest.

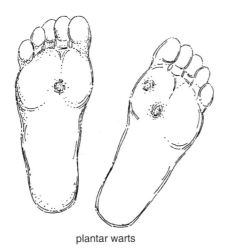

plantar warts

> **Pneumonia**
> Pneumonia is a general term for an infection of the lung. Some forms of pneumonia are:
> *Viral pneumonia.* Early symptoms include sore throat, an achy feeling and a running nose, followed by a cough and fever. Rest and over-the-counter medications to relieve the symptoms are usually adequate treatment.
> *Bacterial pneumonia.* This more serious type of pneumonia usually begins suddenly, with fever

(sometimes up to 104°F or higher), chills, chest pain, shortness of breath and a cough. Later, the cough may produce a blood-streaked mucus. Antibiotics are needed for treatment.

Legionnaire's disease. This fairly rare disease is caused by bacteria, sometimes carried by an infected air supply. The symptoms include nausea, chills, aches, headache, high fever and chest pain. Antibiotics are needed for treatment.

Pneumocystis carinii. A serious lung infection usually seen in elderly people, or those with impaired immune systems, such as AIDS patients. Symptoms include shortness of breath and a frequent cough. Treatment includes antibiotics and other medications.

Polycystic ovary syndrome (PCOS). A condition of unknown cause, in which fluid-filled cysts appear above or below the surface of the ovaries. The cysts interfere with the normal hormonal production of the ovaries and cause irregular menstrual periods.

Other symptoms of PCOS may include substantial weight gain, acne, and increased hair growth on the face, chest, abdomen, and legs (hirsutism). Treatment by a doctor includes prescribing oral contraceptive pills.

Some women with PCOS worry about their ability to become pregnant since they ovulate irregularly. However, pregnancy can occur, and for those who wish to avoid it, contraceptives must be used. Moreover, hormonal contraceptives such as the birth-control pill may help to restore regular periods and decrease the growth of body hair.

Polymerase chain reaction (PCR). A laboratory technique used to detect cells that contain HIV, the AIDS virus, in its active or inactive form.

Postcoital contraceptive (PCC). *See* Morning after pill.

Postpartum. A period of time following the birth of a baby.

Posture. Body carriage. The way you carry yourself can affect your health. When you stand and walk in an erect position, your spinal column is straight, and the organs in your chest and abdomen are in their correct location.

Posture is equally important while sitting, bending over to pick up something, or carrying a heavy object. Sitting up straight against the back of a chair, for example, is better for you than slumping forward. Similarly, bend your knees when picking up an object from the floor. That way, less strain is placed on your spine. When carrying a heavy object, keep it from pulling you over to one side, to minimize strain on your spine. Poor posture places you at risk of developing lower back pain, as well as shoulder, knee, and other bone, joint, or muscle problems.

Good posture prevents such problems; regular exercise helps to maintain it. If you have posture questions or problems, consult your school health clinic or your doctor.

Pot. Street term for marijuana. *See* Marijuana.

Pregnancy. The condition of carrying a developing baby (fetus) in the womb (uterus) for a period of approximately nine months, until the baby is born.

Pregnancy occurs in these stages: First, a female's egg is fertilized by a male's sperm and is now called a zygote. Next, the zygote travels to the uterus. If conditions there are favorable, the zygote settles (implants) in the lining of the uterus. It starts to divide and multiply, and it begins to grow. It is now called an embryo. The first three months of pregnancy are known as the first trimester. After the first trimester, the rapidly growing embryo is called a fetus.

The fetus continues to grow and develop during the next three months (second trimester) and the last three months (third trimester) of pregnancy. After nine months the baby is fully formed and ready to be born.

98

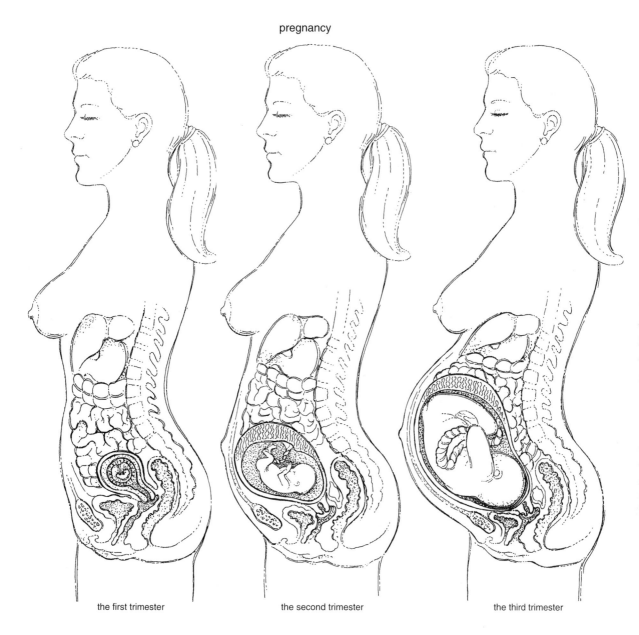

the first trimester the second trimester the third trimester

Pregnancy termination. *See* Abortion.

Pregnancy test. A laboratory procedure to detect the presence of human chorionic gonadotropin (HCG). This hormone is secreted by the placenta, the sac that surrounds, protects, and nourishes the fetus throughout pregnancy. HCG appears in a pregnant woman's blood within a few days after the fertilized egg implants on the uterus wall. It can be detected by a urine test a few days after the first missed menstrual period. A positive test for HCG confirms pregnancy.

Home pregnancy test kits are available in drugstores. However, results should be confirmed by a doctor and a medical examination, since the quality of the home kits varies.

Premature ejaculation. A male's early climax (orgasm, ejaculation) before or shortly after starting the act of sexual intercourse. Premature ejaculation may be a problem for sexual partners: the male may feel sexually incompetent because he cannot control the timing of ejaculation; the female may not be able to reach sexual climax, because females often require more time than men to have an orgasm. Early ejaculation may therefore be a frustrating experience for the female partner. In this situation, the woman may want to reach orgasm through other types of stimulation, such as masturbation.

Many males worry about premature ejaculation, and believe there is nothing they can do to overcome it. However, early ejaculation can be treated with sexual counseling, simple exercises, and the use of a condom to delay ejaculation. Most men can eliminate this worrisome problem after a short period of treatment.

Many young males are concerned about their sexual performance, especially if their friends boast of their abilities. In fact, the average time lapse between erection and ejaculation in adult men is less than five minutes.

Premenstrual syndrome (PMS). A group of physical and emotional changes experienced by some women several days before the start of a period. The changes may include weight gain due to water retention, bloated abdomen, a craving for certain foods, irritability, depression, and other mood changes. The syndrome usually disappears with the onset of the period. If you believe that you have PMS, see your doctor for suggestions on how to relieve your symptoms.

Prenatal care. The medical care and supervision a woman receives during pregnancy. Prenatal care starts with a complete physical checkup at the beginning of pregnancy. This is important for the mother's as well as the developing baby's well-being.

During the first exam the doctor makes sure there are no medical problems that might cause difficulties for the mother or the baby during the pregnancy or after the birth. The mother-to-be also receives advice about nutrition, rest, exercise, and other suggestions for a healthy pregnancy.

A healthy pregnant woman usually continues monthly visits to her doctor, to be certain there are no complications caused by the pregnancy, and that the baby is developing normally. During the last month of pregnancy the mother usually sees her doctor once a week until the baby is born.

Prepuce. *See* Foreskin.

Prevention. Action to forestall development of an illness.

Preventive measures include frequent hand-washing, staying away from someone with a cold, immunization against dangerous childhood diseases, and a healthy lifestyle.

Prophylactic. *See* Condom.

Prophylaxis. A method used to prevent an illness or infection—for example, the use of a condom to avoid acquiring a sexually transmitted disease; or immunization against a contagious disease, such as measles.

Prostaglandins. A group of fatty acids that occur naturally in the body. Prostaglandins perform many functions, including:
- Contraction of smooth muscles, such as those of the uterus
- Regulation of body temperature
- Reduction of blood pressure
- Control of acid secretion in the stomach.

Prostate gland. A male gland located behind the urinary bladder. The prostate gland secretes fluid that becomes a part of a man's ejaculate.

Prostitute. A man or woman who has sex with another person in return for money or other material goods. People who have sex with prostitutes run several major risks, including these:

- Trouble with the law, since prostitution is generally illegal
- Infection, since a prostitute may have one or more sexually transmitted diseases and may transmit them to a healthy client during unprotected sex

Prothrombin time (PT). A blood test to determine the blood's ability to clot in plasma.

Psoriasis. A chronic skin disease that causes dry, flaky, itchy plaques in various body areas. Lesions usually appear on the arms, elbows, chest, and knees. They may last for some time, disappear, and recur at intervals. There is no specific treatment for psoriasis. Medications may be prescribed for itching and other discomfort. They include a wide variety of drugs such as cortisone, anti-inflammatory drugs, and lubricants. Ultraviolet light treatments and exposure to sunlight are often helpful.

Psychoanalysis. *See* Psychotherapy.

Psychopath. A person who has a severe personality disorder, acts in an antisocial manner without regard for others, and may engage in behavior harmful to him-or herself, or to others. A psychopath thinks only about his or her wishes and desires, and is incapable of acting according to conscience.

Psychosis. A state of abnormal behavior in which a person acts inappropriately, because he or she cannot tell the difference between a real situation and one that is wrongly imagined to be true. As a result, the psychotic person may become violent, or behave irrationally without any apparent reason. Psychosis may be caused by a severe biochemical disturbance, by certain illnesses, by drugs, and by drug abuse.

A psychotic person has a severe illness that may require hospitalization for his or her protection as well as for that of others. A psychiatrist must diagnose the nature of the psy-chosis, and prescribe psychotherapy and medications as needed.

Psychosomatic illness. An illness caused by a psychological problem or disorder. Although the cause of the illness is psychological, the symptoms are physical, for example, a headache or a stomachache. To overcome these symptoms, the psychological problem needs to be explored and treated by a mental health professional.

Psychotherapy. Treatment given by a psychologist or psychiatrist to persons who have an emotional disorder. One form of psychotherapy is psychoanalysis, a lengthy process in which a person's mental state is explored during many sessions with a mental health professional. Psychological problems that arose during childhood and later are explored and allowed to come to the surface, so they can be discussed and solved.

More often, psychotherapy is given for a few weeks to a few months, covering a current problem. Another type of psychotherapy is crisis intervention, effective for people suddenly confronted by a major problem, such as the death of a loved one. Still other psychotherapy methods aim to help people by suggesting ways to cope with a particular problem, or by setting goals for behavioral changes that may allow for a more normal way of life.

Puberty. A period of many changes (from age nine to age sixteen) in a person's development from childhood to adolescence. *See also* Tanner stages. These changes involve an increase in the production of various hormones, which cause:

- An increase in height and weight
- Growth of body hair
- Development of breast tissue in girls
- Onset of menstrual bleeding in girls
- Enlargement of the penis and testicles in boys

Pubic hair. Hair around, below, and above the genitals in males and females. Growth of pubic hair is one of the signs of developing physical and sexual maturity. *See also* Puberty.

Pubic lice. *See* Lice, pubic.

Pubis. The bones that make up the front of the pelvis, located in the lowest part of the abdomen. *See illustration* The Human Body.

Pulled muscle. *See* Muscle, pulled.

Pulmonary function tests. A series of tests that measure how well the lungs perform in different situations—for instance, during exercise and during exposure to a variety of environmental factors. The tests also show how well the lungs respond to different medications.

Pulse, taking the. The pulse indicates the heartbeat, its strength, and its rhythm. It is checked by placing the tips of two or three fingers (not the thumb, which has its own pulse) on a point over an artery located close to the body's surface. The best place is just inside the wrist, above the thumb, or under the angle formed where the jawbone meets the neck.

Use a watch with a secondhand, and count the pulse for one minute. The range for the pulse rate varies from 60 to 120 or more beats per minute, depending on a person's age, activity, and state of health.

Babies have a normal pulse rate of 120 to 140, while the adult pulse rate generally ranges from 60 to 80. Pulse rates vary with activity: faster during exercise, slower while at rest. Excitement and stress increase the pulse rate, as does a fever. Depending on a person's state of health, the pulse may be strong or weak, and the pulse rate may be regular or irregular.

Purified protein derivative (PPD). A protein derived from the cell wall of the killed organism that causes tuberculosis. PPD is used to test for the presence of tuberculosis. A small amount is injected under the skin. A red, hardened, or elevated area developing at the injection site within forty-eight hours confirms that the person has been exposed to tuberculosis. *See also* Tuberculosis.

Purpura. A purplish, blotchy condition that appears on various areas of the skin. It is caused by tiny amounts of bleeding. Purpura may develop in response to an infection. It may also be a sign that the person does not have enough blood platelets (tiny solid component particles that help blood to clot).

Pus. The yellow-white fluid that forms in infected body tissues, made up of remnants of bacteria and other foreign particles, and dead white blood cells that attacked the infectious agent.

Q

QNS (Quantity not sufficient). A laboratory abbreviation explaining that the amount of urine, blood, or tissue sample is too small to allow examination.

Quaalude. A "downer" drug that has a calming effect and induces sleep. Quaaludes are habit forming; increased amounts are needed over time to achieve the same effect. Consuming a large dose can be fatal.

Quarantine. Isolation and confinement, used to prevent the spread of a contagious disease. A quarantined infectious person is confined to one place until the infectious period is over. During that time the individual cannot leave the place and cannot receive visitors except health care workers, or persons immune to the disease.

R

Radiation therapy. Use of X rays, radioactive and other radiant energy substances, to treat a variety of diseases, including cancer.

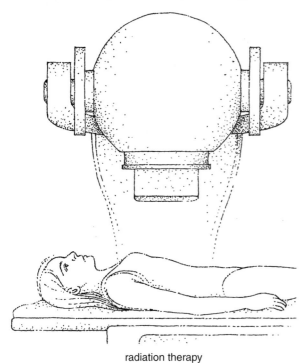

radiation therapy

Radioallergosorbent assay (RAST). A blood test to detect allergy to various chemicals or substances—for example, shrimp, ragweed, and penicillin. *See also* Allergy.

Radioimmunoassay (RIA). A blood test used to determine the quantity of a thyroid hormone or other hormones in the bloodstream.

Radiology. The use of X rays, radioactive substances, or other forms of radiant energy to diagnose and treat a variety of diseases.

Radionuclide scan. A procedure used to study the structure or function of the brain and to detect abnormalities or tumors in

other body areas. A radioactive chemical is injected into a vein. A special (rectilinear or scintillation) camera is used to produce multiple photographs or a videotape, which can then be analyzed for diagnostic purposes.

Rape. A form of sexual assault in which one person forces another to engage in sexual intercourse against her or his will. *See also* Statutory rape.

Guidelines for helping a rape victim
- Report the crime. Help the victim contact the police, or call the police yourself.
- Call a rape hotline, or a friend or relative of the victim for help.
- Contact a doctor or the nearest hospital.
- If the victim has injuries that require immediate attention, turn to Appendix F: First Aid for treatment procedures.
- To help the police identify the attacker, the rape victim should not:
    change clothing
    shower
    brush his or her teeth

Rapid eye movement (REM). Periods of eye activity that occur five to six times during sleep and amount to twenty to twenty-five percent of the total sleep time. During a REM period:
- Respirations are faster and deeper than during non-REM times
- Muscle tone is less active
- Dreams occur
- Some males may have an erection

Rapid plasma reagin test (RPR). A blood test to detect syphilis, a sexually transmitted disease. *See* Syphilis.

Rash. A change in the color, appearance, or texture of an area of skin. A rash may make a skin area appear rough or raised. Depending on the cause, some rashes result in no other symptoms, while others produce itching and burning. Causes include allergy, infection, and direct contact with an irritating substance. Consult a doctor if the rash persists. Treatment depends on the cause of the rash.

Raynaud's disease. A circulatory problem that affects the fingers or toes. These parts may become extremely cold, and sometimes blue, because of excessive sensitivity to cold temperatures of the small arteries that supply blood to the extremities. The arteries' sensitivity to cold and other factors cause them to narrow and go into spasms, reducing blood flow to the fingers and toes. Raynaud's disease is often associated with other conditions or diseases, such as autoimmune disease.

Anyone with this condition should wear warm, loose-fitting gloves and shoes, especially when working or playing in cool or cold weather, and should try to avoid exposure to cold temperatures. When exposure is unavoidable, protective clothing is essential. Other treatment includes attention to the underlying illness, and medication to dilate the narrowed blood vessels.

Rebelliousness, adolescent. Conflict between a teenager's thoughts, wishes, and expectations, and those of parents and other authority figures such as teachers.

Rectum. The lowest part of the intestine. *See illustration* The Human Body; Digestive system.

Recurrent. Happening again and again, or reappearing, as a recurrent illness or symptom.

Red blood cell (rbc). A solid cellular component in blood, produced by the bone marrow. Blood contains millions of red blood cells, which carry hemoglobin. *See* Hemoglobin. In turn, hemoglobin contains oxygen needed by body tissues. As the red blood cells circulate, they carry oxygen to nourish body tissues and they pick up carbon dioxide, the tissues' waste material. When the waste-carrying blood reaches the lungs, carbon dioxide is removed, and new oxygen is picked up. The cycle of cell nourishment and waste removal is repeated several thousand times in each twenty-four-hour period. *See also* Blood.

Refraction. An examination used by an eye specialist (ophthalmologist or optometrist) to determine the need for eyeglasses, and the strength of the lenses required to improve vision.

Rejection (of tissue). The body's immune system, in trying to protect the body against foreign invaders, may attack a skin graft or other transplanted tissue, such as a kidney or heart transplant, from a donor whose tissues do not match those of the recipient. Tissue rejection may be prevented by giving the patient certain medications, called immunosuppressives, which interfere with the immune system's ability to recognize and attack foreign substances.

Rejection, personal. Refusal of one person to accept friendship or love offered by another. This may be a painful experience for the person who is rejected. Still, rejection is a learning experience. Everyone is rejected at one time or another. Often what one person wants or enjoys does not please the other.

A rejected teen should never assume that he or she is worthless because a relationship is not working out. Rejection only means that the two people are not a good match at this time.

Relationship. A friendship in which two people get to know each other well, share experiences, and confide in each other. In a successful relationship, friends become very close, help each other, and share many interests. Although a close relationship may develop into a sexual relationship, many teens have satisfying relationships that do not include sex.

Relaxation exercises. Techniques to help people overcome nervousness, tension, and anxiety. Physical exercise—walking, running, swimming, or bicycling—may help you to feel more relaxed. Meditation, which involves sitting quietly and concentrating on one particular thought or phrase for some time, is another helpful relaxation technique.

Meditation is even more effective when combined with deep, regular breathing and total body muscle relaxation. Try it: Starting with your head, relax the muscles in your face and neck, then those around your shoulders, in your arms, trunk, and legs. Breathe slowly and deeply as your muscles begin to relax. If you do this for ten to twenty minutes, your whole body will feel relaxed and free of tension.

In another relaxation technique, imagine you are in a restful, pleasant place—for example, at the beach or near a lake. The sun is shining, the sky is blue, and waves gently lap at the shore. Concentrate on these pleasurable thoughts to help your body to relax and to reduce tension or anxiety.

REM. *See* Rapid eye movement.

Remission. A period of time in which a person with a chronic illness such as cancer has no symptoms of the disease.

Repetitive stress injury (RSI). A group of medical problems caused by certain motions or activities performed over and over again, perhaps at work (typing, sorting mail) or during sports (pitching a ball). Such activities, done incorrectly or over long periods of time, can cause pain, stiffness, numbness, weakness, and other symptoms.

Treatment includes Rest, Ice, Compression, and Elevation (RICE) of the affected body part . Medication may be needed to relieve pain and inflammation. In severe cases, a brace or surgery may be required.

Reproductive system, female. The organs that enable a woman to menstruate, have sex, carry a pregnancy, give birth to a baby, and produce breast milk to nourish it.

The female reproductive system consists of the breasts, ovaries, fallopian tubes, uterus, cervix, and vagina. Glands located in the brain secrete hormones that regulate the functions of the reproductive system, such as the onset of puberty and menstruation. The same glands and others also help to prepare the uterus for pregnancy and stimulate the breasts of a new mother to secrete milk (lactation). *See* illustration, page 106.

Reproductive system, male. The organs that function to produce sexual potency, sperm, and semen. The male system includes the testicles, the ducts that carry semen from each testicle (epididymis and vas deferens), and the penis. Certain glands in the brain secrete hormones that stimulate the sex drive and the production of sperm, which is discharged from the penis during sexual intercourse. *See* illustration, page 107.

Rescue breathing. *See* Appendix F: First Aid.

Respirations. Respirations indicate the functioning of the lungs as a person breathes in (inspirations), and breathes out (expirations), bringing oxygen into the body, and expelling carbon dioxide. Average normal respiratory rates range from fifteen to eighteen respirations per minute and in babies, from forty to fifty per minute.

Respiratory rates vary with activity and state of health. They increase during exercise or stress, and decrease when a person is at rest. Many circumstances can cause variations in the respiratory rate. A person with a high fever or certain illnesses, for example, may have a higher than normal rate, while a sleeping person may have a slower rate.

To measure respirations: Time the rise and fall of the chest for one minute, prefer-

the female reproductive system (front)

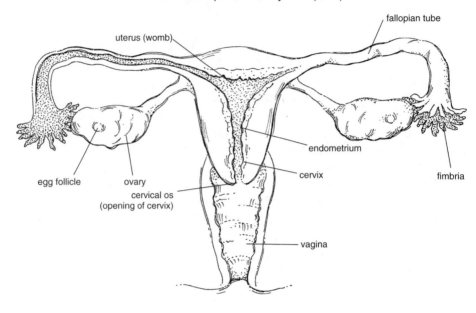

uterus (womb)

fallopian tube

egg follicle

ovary

cervical os
(opening of cervix)

endometrium

cervix

fimbria

vagina

the female reproductive system (side)

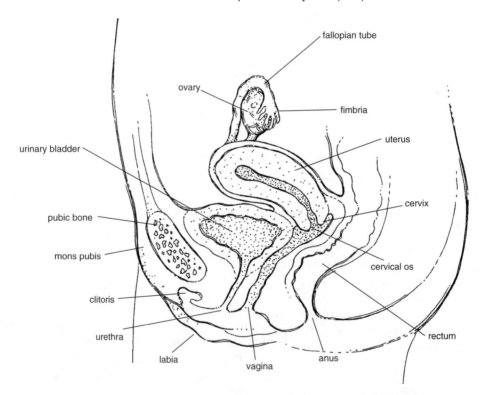

fallopian tube

ovary

fimbria

uterus

urinary bladder

cervix

pubic bone

mons pubis

cervical os

clitoris

urethra

labia

vagina

anus

rectum

the male reproductive system (front)

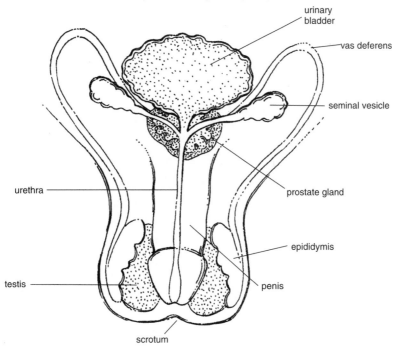

urinary bladder

vas deferens

seminal vesicle

prostate gland

epididymis

penis

urethra

testis

scrotum

the male reproductive system (side)

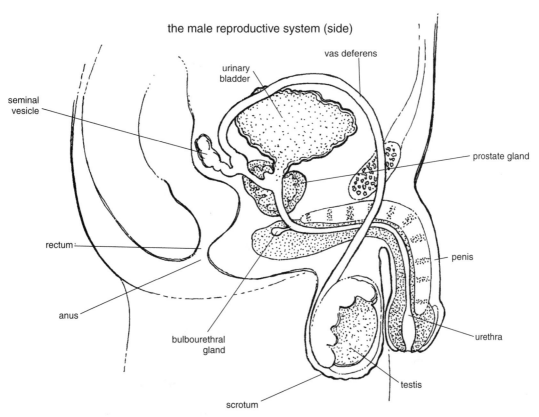

vas deferens

urinary bladder

seminal vesicle

prostate gland

rectum

penis

anus

bulbourethral gland

urethra

testis

scrotum

ably while the person is sleeping or not paying attention to you. The reason to choose this time is that emotional changes, such as fear, anxiety, or excitement, affect the respiratory rate and may cause an inaccurate reading.

Respiratory distress syndrome (RDS). Inadequate functioning of the heart and lungs, preventing the essential exchange of oxygen and carbon dioxide. The result is potentially life-threatening difficulty in breathing.

RDS may be caused by a toxic reaction to certain chemicals or drugs, severe infection, lung injury, near-drowning, or accidental entry of food into the lungs (aspiration).

RDS requires immediate hospitalization and treatment to save the patient's life, especially if the onset is sudden (acute respiratory distress syndrome, ARDS).

Retardation, mental. Slow, below-average ability to understand or learn. A person may be retarded as a result of certain infections or illnesses acquired before, during, or shortly after birth, or because of illnesses contracted during early childhood. A retarded child has difficulty in following regular class work and may need special classes. A retarded adult may be able to live and work in a special environment, such as a supervised group home, or a workshop for people with such handicaps.

Retina. The inner layer (lining) of the eyeball. The retina serves as a focusing center for light rays coming through the lens of the eye, and transmits the image to the brain by way of electrical signals.

Retina, detached. A serious condition in which the retina is separated from the other layers of the eyeball. This may happen as a result of trauma or certain types of eye surgery, or in persons who are very nearsighted. Surgery may be needed to prevent partial or complete loss of vision in the affected eye.

Retrograde ejaculation. Ejaculate that flows backward toward the bladder instead of toward the penis. Some teens achieve retrograde ejaculation by holding the opening of the penis closed so it cannot discharge the ejaculate after they masturbate or have sex. Retrograde ejaculation may cause the prostate gland to swell up and become painful or infected.

Retroverted uterus. A womb that is tipped backward toward the spine. The uterus may change its position without causing any problems. However, if the backward-tipped position causes pain or other complaints during periods or at other times, a pelvic examination is needed to find the cause. Treatment is then given as needed.

Reye's syndrome. A disorder that may occur in a child after contracting a viral disease, for example, chickenpox or influenza. The cause is unknown. Aspirin appears to play some part in the development of Reye's syndrome, and therefore should not be given to a child ill with a respiratory or other minor illness that includes fever.

Early symptoms of Reye's syndrome are vomiting and drowsiness. If the condition remains unrecognized, major organs such as the brain, kidneys, and the liver are affected. The child may become unconscious, or develop seizures. Other internal changes occur, and the child may die if not treated promptly.

A child with Reye's syndrome must be hospitalized for life-saving treatment. This includes administration of intravenous fluids to normalize the composition of the blood, medications, and other measures that prevent swelling of the brain, reduction of elevated temperature, and immediate care to deal with other symptoms as they arise.

Rheumatic heart disease. A heart condition that may develop in children or teens who receive inadequate or no treatment for streptococcal infections such as scarlet fever, strep throat, or tonsillitis. During the acute stage of such a disease, a youngster may have a high fever and inflammation of the lining of the heart and valves. Wrist, ankle, and knee joints may also become inflamed and painful. Treatment includes bed rest, anti-inflammatory drugs, and good nutrition.

If this condition is not treated, attacks of joint pain may recur at intervals. The heart valves may heal but may become thickened with scar tissue, which interferes with the normal heart functioning. Lifelong heart damage may result.

Rheumatoid arthritis (RA). Swelling, inflammation, and pain in the joints of the fingers, wrists, knees, and toes that may damage the joints and cause disability. The cause of RA is unknown; it may be due to an abnormality of the immune system.

Treatment includes medications to relieve pain and decrease inflammation and swelling of the affected joints. Exercise is important: it can decrease stiffness in the joints and keep them flexible, allowing for better mobility.

Rheumatoid factor (RF). A substance found in the blood of persons who have certain conditions such as rheumatoid arthritis.

Rh factor. A substance found in the blood of 85 percent of Americans; these individuals are said to be Rh positive. Those who do not have the Rh factor in their blood are Rh negative. Pregnant women and persons who need blood transfusions must be tested to determine their Rh status. The test is done before administering any blood, to make sure an Rh-negative person does not receive Rh-positive blood. This could cause a serious adverse reaction.

An Rh-negative woman who is pregnant by an Rh-positive man faces a different danger. If she is not treated within seventy-two hours after having a miscarriage or abortion, or giving birth to an Rh-positive baby, she may develop antibodies that will harm her next baby. The second baby may be born with a serious blood disease (erythroblastosis fetalis). Treatment with RhoGAM, an immune globulin substance, prevents this potentially fatal condition.

Rhinoplasty. Plastic reconstructive surgery of the nose, performed to repair damage caused by a defect or injury, or to improve the shape of the nose.

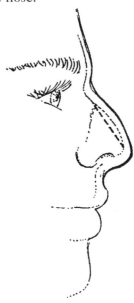

rhinoplasty

Rhythm method. A form of birth control. A woman who uses this method abstains from having sex during days 8 to 16 (the middle) of her menstrual cycle. During these days, the ovary releases an egg (ovulation), which travels to the uterus. If the woman has sex during this time, sperm may penetrate the egg and cause pregnancy.

The rhythm method can prevent pregnancy if a woman finds the exact time of ovulation during each menstrual cycle and avoids having sex during that time, and during the five to six days before ovulation. This is how the rhythm method works:

- The woman takes her temperature every day during the menstrual cycle to determine her time of ovulation
- When she notes a slight rise in temperature (the sign that she is ovulating), she avoids having sex for several days
- The egg can now travel to the uterus without meeting any sperm
- The uterus discards the unfertilized egg during her next period
- No pregnancy occurs

If a woman uses the rhythm method every month and avoids having sex during the time of ovulation, she may be able to prevent a pregnancy. Unfortunately, this method is not totally reliable because ovulation times vary from one month to the next, and many teens have irregular periods. It is therefore not always possible to know when to avoid sex and so prevent pregnancy.

The Pill, condom, and diaphragm, when used correctly, provide a higher rate of protection against pregnancy than the rhythm method.

Ribonucleic acid. *See* RNA.

RICE. An acronym for rest, ice, compression, and elevation, the treatment recommended for muscle strains and other sports injuries.

Ringworm. An infectious skin disease caused by a fungus (no worm is involved), which produces a ring-shaped rash. Ringworm may appear on the scalp or in other body areas. Antifungal medication is the treatment.

Risk reduction. A process to decrease your chances of an accident, injury, or infection. By thinking and planning ahead and by learning about various risks, you can protect yourself in potentially harmful situations. High-risk situations involve:

Alcohol and substance abuse. You can reduce the risks of many physical and mental

the RICE treatment for sports injuries

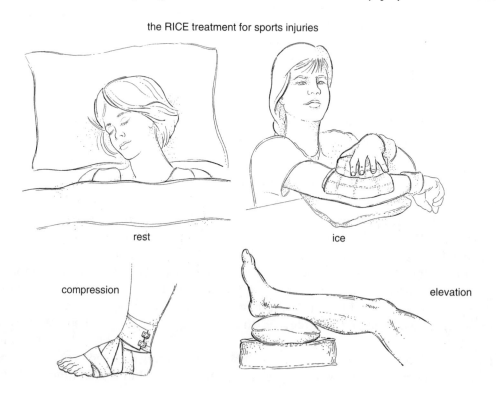

rest

ice

compression

elevation

problems by not using alcohol or dangerous street drugs.

Pregnancy. You can reduce the risk of pregnancy by not having sex or by avoiding unprotected sex. A condom, diaphragm, or other contraceptive methods, used exactly as instructed, will reduce the risk.

A pregnant female can reduce the risks of pregnancy and contribute to her infant's safe delivery and good health by receiving prenatal care at an early stage in the pregnancy.

Sports injuries. You can reduce the risk of a sports injury by following the coach's instructions and by avoiding excessive exercise and sports activities.

Sexually transmitted diseases, HIV infection, AIDS. A few precautions will greatly reduce your risk of contracting sexually transmitted diseases (STDs), HIV infection, and AIDS. The most important ones are:

- Be aware that any sex partner may have one or more sexually transmitted infections or be infected with HIV and may pass the infection on to you. Know the health status (including drug habits) and sexual history of a sex partner.
- Drug and alcohol use expose you to risks. They may impair your judgment. Under the influence of drugs or alcohol, you may be more likely to have sex with an infected partner.
- Do not participate in unprotected sex. Use a condom that contains nonoxynol-9, a chemical agent that provides a high degree of protection against infection and pregnancy.

RNA (ribonucleic acid). RNA and DNA (deoxyribonucleic acid) are molecules present in every living cell. Together, RNA and DNA carry and transmit each characteristic or trait passed on by living beings to their offspring. *See also* DNA.

***Roe v. Wade* decision.** A case decided by the U.S. Supreme Court that gives women the right to obtain an abortion. Some states have placed limits on this right by modifying the decision, depending on the age and circumstances of the woman who wants the abortion and on other factors.

Rotator cuff injury. Inflammation or tearing of the muscles that surround the shoulder area. Treatment includes rest, application of ice, exercise, and, occasionally, surgery.

RU-486. An oral drug, now being used in the United States in experimental studies only, that brings about an abortion if given very early during pregnancy (within three weeks after the first missed menstrual period). RU-486 causes strong uterine contractions, which expel the embryo and terminate the pregnancy. The drug is not currently available in this country.

Rubber. Condom.

Rubella (German measles). *See* Measles, German.

Rubeola. *See* Measles.

Safe sex. Sexual relations free of any risk of contracting HIV or other sexually transmitted infections. Safe sex is possible only when both partners are known to be free of infection, as in a long-term monogamous relationship, such as marriage. In a casual relationship, sex is never completely safe even if some form of protection is used, because no protective device is 100 percent effective. Under these circumstances, the only safe sex is no sex.

Safer sex. Sexual relations or activities performed while using protection such as a condom or diaphragm and spermicidal jelly. Although no device will guarantee safety, protected sex reduces the risk of disease.

Salmonella. A microscopic organism (bacterium) that causes severe, often life-threatening intestinal infection. Salmonella infection occurs when foods are not properly cooked, stored, or refrigerated. Summer is the riskiest season, when food may be left out in warm temperatures, allowing the Salmonella organisms to grow and multiply. This is a special hazard at picnics.

To prevent Salmonella infection, perishable foods such as meat, fish, mayonnaise, and dairy foods must be refrigerated at all times. Washing hands before handling food, to remove Salmonella organisms present on the skin, also helps prevent contamination. *See also* Food poisoning.

Salpingitis. Inflammation of the fallopian tubes, which extend—one on either side—from the uterus. *See also* Reproductive system, female.

Saltpeter. Potassium nitrate, a chemical. In earlier times this substance was believed to reduce the sex drive.

Sanitary napkin. A pad made of cotton material, worn externally to absorb the menstrual flow during menstrual periods.

Satyriasis. *See* Nymphomania.

Scabies. A skin condition spread during sexual or other direct contact with an infected person.

Cause: A tiny insectlike creature (mite) that burrows into the skin.

Symptoms: Severe itching, small itchy blisters and other skin lesions topped by a pin-sized blood crust, and scratch marks. Burrows appear as slightly elevated gray marks where mites have entered the skin. Lesions occur on the hands, breasts, genitals, and other body parts.

Treatment: All family members, even those without symptoms, must follow these steps:

- Take a shower
- Apply Elimite cream to cover the body from the neck to the tips of the toes; leave medication on for three to four hours
- After four hours, complete treatment with another shower or bath
- Wash all clothing, sheets, and towels in hot water, or have them dry-cleaned
- Hang jackets, coats, and other outerwear in a closed closet and leave them for two weeks. This will kill the mites, which

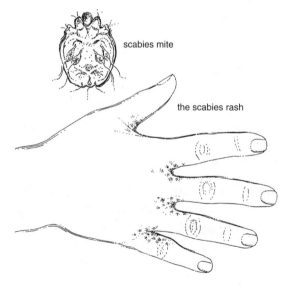

scabies mite

the scabies rash

can't survive without a meal of blood. Small children, pregnant women, and nursing mothers may require other forms of treatment, to prevent lengthy exposure to the chemical in the medication and possible harm to the fetus or baby.

Complications: Additional infection caused by scratching.

Sexual precautions: No sex for at least forty-eight hours after treatment is completed.

Scan. *See* CT scan; Radionuclide scan.

Schizophrenia. A type of psychosis (mental illness) in which a person is unable to tell the difference between a real situation and one that is pure fantasy. The cause of the disease is not well understood, but may be due to biochemical changes that occur during adolescence or early adult life.

Schizophrenia is a dangerous mental disease. A schizophrenic person may have hallucinations (see things and situations that are not there), hear voices that command the performance of certain acts that may cause harm to others or the sick person, and be unable to think logically or follow a conversation. Treatment consists of hospitalization, psychotherapy, drugs that control the psychosis (antipsychotic drugs), and rehabilitation programs that help the sick person resume a normal life.

Although a person may recover from the disease, recurrences are possible.

Scoliosis. A deformity of the spine, which may curve sideways or look S-shaped. Spinal curvature often develops during the early teen years or even earlier.

Mild curvature is treated by prescribed exercises. If the curvature becomes more severe, a metal rod is surgically implanted in the back to keep the spine straight. A cast may be applied and worn by the patient for some time to maintain correct spinal posture.

Scrotum. A pouchlike sac underneath the

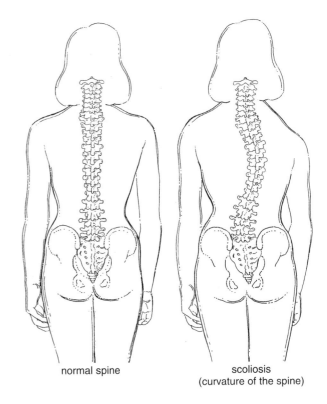

normal spine

scoliosis
(curvature of the spine)

penis. The sac holds the testicles. *See illustration* The Human Body.

Sebaceous cyst. A small sac under the skin filled with sebum, an oily fluid secreted by the sebaceous glands. *See also* Cyst; Sebum.

Sebaceous gland. A skin gland that secretes sebum, an oily substance that prevents dry skin.

Seborrheic dermatitis. An oily skin condition caused by excess oil production. The condition may cause dandruff (dead skin cells on the scalp). *See also* Dermatitis; Contact dermatitis.

Sebum. An oily substance secreted by the sebaceous glands.

Secondary amenorrhea. Delay of a menstrual period by more than six weeks in a woman who has previously menstruated. Secondary amenorrhea may be caused by hormonal irregularity or by various illnesses. A medical examination is necessary to determine the cause and the appropriate treatment. *See also* Amenorrhea.

Secondary dysmenorrhea. Discomfort during menstruation, caused by illness, a growth, or an infection. A medical examination is needed to diagnose the cause and determine proper treatment. *See also* Dysmenorrhea.

Secondary infection. Infection that follows an earlier infection. For example, a person may have the flu, a viral infection that weakens the immune system. Bacteria may then be able to start an additional, or secondary, infection, such as pneumonia.

Secondary virginity. *See* Virgin.

Seizure. Sudden muscle spasms that may range from mild to severe. A seizure is caused by abnormalities in the brain's nerve cells that lead to abnormal electrical discharges. A person having a seizure may become temporarily unconscious, lose bladder control, and later be unable to remember what happened. Mild (petit mal) seizures may not cause muscle spasms. The person may be found staring into space, unaware of the surroundings. This type of seizure may last only a few seconds; but if it occurs several times a day, it interferes with normal life activities.

Infants running a high fever sometimes have a seizure. Certain illnesses such as epilepsy may cause seizures from time to time. A brain tumor, certain drugs, and sudden stopping of long-term heavy alcohol use may also cause seizures. *See also* Appendix F: First Aid, Seizures.

Self-esteem, self-respect. A person's confident feeling that he or she can deal with life's challenges. Self-esteem is important for anyone, but especially for teens preparing for adult life.

Teens with little or no self-esteem may become depressed—unhappy about how they feel about themselves and dissatisfied with their ability to face life. This dissatisfaction may make them feel worthless, especially if they have few friends. Some may believe they don't deserve to have friends.

A teen who has poor self-esteem needs help. If you have this problem, don't wait: ask to see a counselor right away. It's important to discover the reason for these feelings and to get help for this serious problem.

Self-examination. *See* Breast self-examination; Testicular self-examination.

Self-image. What and how you think of yourself. If your self-image is positive, you think well of yourself and your accomplishments, and you have many different interests.

A person with a negative self-image may think he or she has few abilities and social skills. Teens who have a negative self-image often feel unattractive and unworthy of friendship or love. Causes of a poor self-image include rejection by a friend, troubled family relationships, low grades, and poor performance in sports. Any teen with such negative feelings needs help quickly. He or she should see a doctor, counselor, or member of the clergy. *See also* Self-esteem.

Semen, ejaculate. Fluid containing sperm. Semen is stored in the seminal vesicles (above the prostate gland) and discharged in the ejaculate during sexual climax. *See illustration* The Human Body.

Semen analysis. A laboratory test to determine the quality and possible deficiencies of semen. To obtain a semen sample, the man masturbates and deposits the ejaculate into a sterile container. The semen is measured and examined under a microscope. Sperm are counted and examined for appearance and motion. If the sperm count is low, or if the sperm are deformed or move very slowly, the man may have difficulty starting a pregnancy in his female partner.

Seminal fluid. Fluid secreted by the prostate and other glands. The fluid carries semen out of the male's body.

Seminal vesicles. Two saclike glands near a male's prostate and bladder. They secrete fluid and store sperm.

Septum, deviated. *See* Deviated septum.

Sequential multiple analysis (SMA, Chem screen). A blood test that analyzes many biochemical constituents of blood in a specific sequence.

Seroconversion. A positive result in blood that tested negative for an infection during an earlier examination.

Sex. A set of characteristics that determines the difference between male and female; also shorthand for "sexual intercourse."

Sex, anal. Sexual activity that involves insertion of one partner's penis into the other partner's rectum. Since the anus produces no lubricating mucus, tears or fissures in the skin may result, allowing for the spread of infection between partners. Use of condoms can help to prevent this spread. The condom must be changed before other sexual activity to prevent infection.

Sex, delayed. Putting off a sexual relationship until a later time in life. Teens spend a lot of time thinking about their sexuality. One of the most important decisions about sex is: when is the time right to start having sex?

A sexual relationship involves personal closeness and physical intimacy. For this reason both partners need to consider whether they are physically and emotionally ready for such a relationship, and able to accept the risks, consequences, and responsibilities involved.

Many teens decide that it is a good idea to delay a sexual relationship until they feel sure that they are ready.

Sex education. Teaching methods developed by specially trained instructors who can explain and discuss the following topics:
- Sexual development, feelings, emotions, and decision making
- Family planning and contraception
- Sexual activities such as intercourse and outercourse
- Unsafe sex, safer sex, safe sex
- The need to respect persons of a different sexual orientation
- The risks and consequences of various sexual activities, and how to avoid them
- Rape, date rape, and other forms of sexual assault
- Sexually transmitted diseases, HIV infection, and AIDS

Sex flush. Reddening of the skin during sexual excitement.

Sex guilt. Uncomfortable feelings about having sexual relations. This unease is usually caused by moral or religious considerations or by a conflict with parents who disapprove of teens having sex.

Teens who have guilt feelings about sex should discuss their feelings with a trusted family member, clergy member, or counselor. Talking it out helps teens to make the decisions about sex that are right for them, and restores comfortable feelings.

Sex, heterosexual. Sexual relations between a man and a woman.

Sex, homosexual. Sexual relations between a man and another man or between a woman and another woman.

Sex, love. Affection and commitment expressed by having sexual relations with a partner, as in marriage.

Sex, misconceptions. False beliefs concerning sex. Examples of false beliefs:
1. "You can't become pregnant when you have sex the first time." *Not true.* You certainly *can* become pregnant during a first sexual encounter.
2. "You can't get pregnant if you have sex while standing up." *Not true.* You *can* get pregnant if you have sex standing up just as easily as if you have sex lying down.

Sex, oral. Sexual activity that involves contact between one partner's mouth and the other partner's genitals.

Sex, protected. Sexual relations while using birth control or other devices intended to prevent pregnancy and sexually transmitted diseases. *See also* Safer sex.

Sex, readiness for. Having the physical and emotional maturity to feel comfortable in a sexual relationship. *See* Sex, delayed.

Sex, safe. *See* Safe sex; Safer sex.

Sex, unprotected. Sexual intercourse without the use of a device or medication to prevent sexually transmitted diseases and pregnancy.

Sexual abuse. *See* Abuse.

Sexual activity, premature. Sexual intercourse by young teens who are not emotionally or physically ready to have sex.

Sexual assault. Sexual activity forced by one person on another against that person's will. *See also* Rape.

Sexual choices. Decisions about how, when, where, with whom, and in what manner to engage in sexual activities. For example, a person may want to show affection and love to a partner, but may not feel ready to have sexual intercourse. Kissing or hugging may be sexual choices that will satisfy both partners at the time.

Sexual desire. Sexual attraction of one person to another.

Sexual fantasies. Pictures in a person's mind of having sex in various situations, places, or positions. Fantasies are the product of imagination, not usually intended to be carried out in real life. A person who actually wants to carry out a fantasy should consider it very carefully.

Most people have sexual fantasies at one time or another. They become a problem only if they take up time needed for studies, work, fun with friends, or sports. If you spend a great deal of time spinning sexual fantasies, consult a doctor, school nurse, or other health professional.

Sexual intercourse, heterosexual. Sexual activity during which a male inserts his penis into a female's vagina. A couple may prepare for sexual intercourse with foreplay. This includes kissing, fondling, or caressing each other. Foreplay increases the sexual pleasure and excitement of both partners and helps the man's penis to become erect.

During sexual intercourse, the man makes thrusting movements with his penis and body until he reaches his sexual climax (orgasm) and ejaculates into the woman's vagina. The woman also makes thrusting movements with her body until she, too, has an orgasm. She may have her orgasm at the same time as her partner, or she may have it later or earlier, or even multiple times. No fluid is released, but there may be a series of involuntary muscle contractions, causing intense pleasure.

Sexuality. Awareness of one's sexual feelings.

Sexually transmitted disease (STD), infection. (Formerly called venereal disease,

VD.) An infection spread to a partner through sexual intercourse or some other sexual activity. Syphilis and gonorrhea are two sexually transmitted diseases. *See* entries for specific diseases.

Sexual stimulation. Use of affectionate speech or physical activities such as kissing, fondling, or caressing to arouse or increase a partner's sexual desire. *See also* Foreplay.

Shingles (herpes zoster). A virus infection caused by one type of herpes virus. The virus affects nerve endings in the skin in one or several body areas; blisters and crusty lesions then develop along the affected nerve paths.

Shingles can be very painful. The infection usually lasts several weeks or longer. The drug acyclovir (Zovirax), also used for other types of herpes infections, is the treatment for shingles.

Shin splints. Pain in the front portion of the large, weight-bearing shinbone (tibia), caused by tiny tears in the soft tissues that cover the bone. Shin splints often occur as a result of frequent jogging or running on hard surfaces, especially without well-cushioned athletic shoes.

To prevent shin splints: (1) avoid running on hard pavement, and run or jog instead on soft surfaces such as grass, sand, or a school track; (2) wear good-quality, cushioned running shoes with arch supports.

Shock. A reaction by the body to a trauma—such as severe bleeding (hemorrhage), illness, infection, injury, stress, allergy, burn, or other major event—that causes failure of the circulatory system and collapse, unless promptly treated and reversed. Symptoms of shock include weakness; pale, cold, moist skin; irregular, shallow breathing; rapid pulse; nausea; low blood pressure; and insufficient amounts of urine. Shock may not occur immediately after onset of the trauma, but may develop later (delayed shock).

Immediate first aid for shock includes:
- Call for an ambulance
- Have the person lie down, and lower the head to a level below the feet, provided there is no head or chest injury
- Stop any bleeding
- Loosen clothing to ease breathing
See also Appendix F: First Aid.

Further treatment depends on the cause. Shock caused by:
- *Bleeding* is treated with blood transfusions to replace lost blood
- *Fluid loss* is treated with intravenous replacement of fluids
- *Illness or infection* is treated with drugs and other measures specific for these conditions
- *Anaphylaxis (anaphylactic shock),* caused by extreme allergic reaction, is treated with injections of drugs that reverse the reaction
- *Contact with electric current* is treated by separating the person from the current, then providing treatment to restore heart and respiratory function. *Caution:* Before touching the person, turn off the current, if possible, to protect yourself. If not possible, use a dry, nonconducting object (wooden plank, chair, broomstick) to separate the person from the current.
- *Lightning strike* requires basic treatment for shock and to restore heartbeat and breathing. A person struck by lightning does not conduct electricity and may be touched without risk.
- *Severe burn* requires basic treatment for shock, and other treatment measures depending on the nature of the burn, which may be caused by heat or a chemical substance
- *Insulin shock,* an excessively low blood sugar level in a person who has diabetes, is treated with intravenous glucose to raise the blood sugar to a normal level
- *Diabetic coma,* caused by an excessively

high blood sugar level in a person who has diabetes, is treated with intravenous administration of insulin to lower blood sugar to normal

All forms of shock, whatever the cause, are serious and may become life-threatening if not treated promptly. A person in shock must be hospitalized for intensive treatment and monitoring to reverse shock and restore normal body function. *See also* Appendix F: First Aid, Shock.

Shock, emotional. An intense reaction to an unexpected event that causes a strong positive or negative response.

Shock therapy. *See* Electroshock therapy.

Sickle-cell disease. An inherited illness that primarily affects African-Americans. Children born with this disease have sickle-shaped red blood cells, which may produce serious problems in blood circulation.

The sickle shape of the red blood cells causes blood clots in the cells, which then hinder the normal flow of blood. Sickle cells are fragile and may be destroyed while circulating. Symptoms of sickle-cell disease include anemia, arthritislike joint pains, and infections in various body areas. Treatment

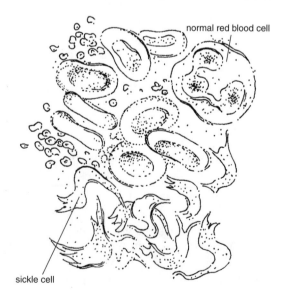

normal red blood cell

sickle cell

focuses on specific symptoms. *See also* Sickle-cell trait.

Sickle-cell trait. An abnormal blood cell condition. A blood test shows some sickle-shaped blood cells, mixed with normal, oval red blood cells. A person with sickle-cell trait has no symptoms and lives a normal life. Genetic counseling is important for a couple considering having children if they know or suspect that one partner has sickle-cell trait. The genetic counselor will explain the potential risk of having a child born with sickle-cell trait or sickle-cell disease. *See also* Sickle-cell disease.

Sigmoidoscopy. *See* Endoscopy.

Sinus. A hollow cavity somewhere in the body; for example, a hollow space in a bone. A sinus may also be a channel for the passage of blood or lymph fluid. Finally, a sinus may develop following an infection.

Sinusitis. Inflammation of the lining of a sinus, most commonly in the paranasal sinuses (inside the bones above and around the nose). The cause is usually a bacterial or viral infection which prevents the normal drainage of fluid into and out of the nose.

Treatment involves drinking large quantities of fluids, the use of a vaporizer, and a decongestant to clear clogged nasal passages by shrinking the swollen mucous membranes. Antibiotics may be prescribed to fight the infection.

Skin, problems. Abnormal conditions of the body's protective covering. Exposure to various substances inside or outside the body may cause a rash, blisters, or other abnormal skin conditions. Dry or excessively oily skin may lead to problems such as acne. Certain illnesses and infections may cause a rash, skin discoloration, or other problems.

If you notice a change in your skin, see your doctor. You need to find out the reason for the change so you can take care of the underlying problem. *See also* Acne, Contact dermatitis; Seborrheic dermatitis.

Skin tests. Tests done by an allergist (specialist in allergy problems) to determine the substances or organisms to which a person may be allergic. Common causes of allergies include pollen, grass, dust, and dander from animals such as cats and dogs.

The allergist injects a small amount of extract from a suspected substance (allergen) under the skin and then observes the reaction. An itchy red blotch that appears at the injection site within twenty minutes confirms an allergy to that substance.

The allergist can then develop a treatment plan involving a series of injections of tiny amounts of the allergy-causing substance. Over time, these injections will build up immunity and desensitize the patient against the substance. *See also* Allergy.

Slipped femoral epiphysis. A condition seen in children and teens, involving weakness, dislocation, and pain in a portion of the thighbone anywhere between the shaft and its gristlelike cover (cartilage).

As a child's or teen's bones grow and develop, the cartilage cover sometimes separates from the bone, causing weakness and pain. This problem may develop at the hip end of the femur (thighbone). It usually occurs in one leg but sometimes affects both.

Slipped femoral epiphysis occurs most often in heavy teens and is seen more frequently in boys than in girls. Early diagnosis and surgery offer the best chance for a complete recovery.

Slit lamp. A device used by an eye doctor to determine certain abnormalities of the eyes.

Smegma. Oily material secreted by glands located in the foreskin of the penis and in the inner lips of the vagina.

Smoking. Using and inhaling tobacco in cigarettes, cigars, or pipes; a harmful but common practice among young people and adults. Tobacco contains nicotine, a toxic substance that causes a rapid heartbeat, dizziness, and nausea.

Physical contact with nicotine—for example, the lips with a cigarette or the throat with inhaled smoke—irritates and damages the respiratory passages, the lungs, and many other organs. Studies show that active smoking can cause cancer and other conditions that affect blood vessels and the heart, leading to progressive, potentially fatal illness.

Passive smoking—being near someone who smokes—produces similar conditions. Nonsmokers may inhale air that is smoke-laden due to nearby smokers.

Sodomy. Anal or oral intercourse with another person.

Sonogram (SONO). A diagnostic method in which sound waves bounce off various tissues and then trace a pictorial pattern. A doctor or other health professional analyzes the picture to see if the tissues are healthy; if not, the picture helps in the diagnosis of the problem.

Spanish fly. An extract made from dried beetles (cantharides). In the past, this substance was used for medical purposes. Some people used Spanish fly as a sexual stimulant. Spanish fly is a highly toxic substance, however, and should not be used for any purpose.

Specimen (spec). A small quantity of urine, blood, or other body fluid or tissue examined for diagnostic purposes.

Speculum. A medical instrument used to examine the interior parts of a woman's vagina and cervix.

Speech defect. Difficulty in clearly forming words or sentences. A child who cannot speak clearly may lisp (be unable to pronounce the "s" sound), stutter (get stuck on one syllable of a word, unable to continue without pausing in mid-word), or have other difficulties in speaking accurately and clearly.

Speech defects may be caused by poor hearing, learning disability, mental retardation, or brain damage. To correct a speech defect, the underlying problem, such as impaired hearing, must be diagnosed and corrected. The speech defect is then treated by a speech pathologist, who examines the child and determines which exercises should be done to allow the mouth and tongue muscles and other structures to make the appropriate sounds needed for correct, clear speech.

Speed. Slang for amphetamine, a stimulant that increases the user's wakefulness, muscle strength, and sense of well-being. This drug is dangerous because the user:
- May become dependent on the drug
- Does not recognize overexertion
- Is unaware of fatigue

Sperm. A tiny, tadpolelike cell that contains male genetic material. Sperm are produced in the testicles. If a sperm unites with a female's egg, and if that fertilized egg settles in the female's uterus, a pregnancy may be started. *See also* Reproductive system, male.

Spermatic cord. *See* Vas deferens.

Spermatocele. A tissue sac (cyst) containing sperm, located on the tube connected to the testicle (epididymis). A urologist (specialist in diseases of the genitourinary tract) can determine if treatment is needed. A small cyst may require no treatment. A large cyst may need to be surgically removed.

Spermicidal. Refers to a sperm-killing substance.

Spermicide. A substance that kills sperm, available as a foam or jelly. Spermicides are usually used with a barrier contraceptive de-

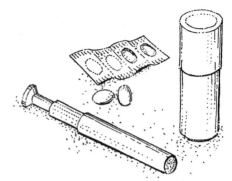

Spermicides are available as creams, jellies, foams, vaginal inserts, and vaginal contraceptive film (VCF), a thin square of absorbable material saturated with a spermicide.

vice such as a condom, diaphragm, sponge, or cervical cap. *See also* Contraceptive.

Spider veins. Tiny blood vessels that appear under the skin on the legs and look like spider-weblike, reddish-blue marks. Spider veins are generally harmless but may be unsightly in large numbers. Injection therapy may be used if a substantial number of spider veins are present.

Spinal fluid. A normally colorless fluid that bathes the brain and spinal cord. A specimen of the fluid is sometimes removed for diagnostic testing.

Spiritual healing. The use of prayer, meditation, and other methods in an effort to restore mental, physical, or emotional health.

Spleen. An organ located in the left upper abdomen. It is part of the lymphatic system, and rids the body of old, worn-out red blood cells. The spleen also helps the body to fight infections. It "coats" bacteria, and so makes it easier for white blood cells to find and destroy them. Some of the spleen's other functions are as yet poorly understood. *See also* Lymphatic system; *illustration* The Human Body.

Sponge, contraceptive. A small polyurethane sponge that contains the spermicide nonoxynol-9 and acts as a barrier contraceptive to prevent pregnancy.

The sponge has been discontinued by the manufacturer due to inability to meet government regulations, but it may still be available in clinics or drugstores, under the name, Today Vaginal Contraceptive Sponge.

The sponge may be inserted in the vagina up to twenty-four hours before intercourse and should be left in place for at least six hours afterward. If intercourse is repeated, no further spermicide is needed during this six-hour period. *See also* Contraceptive.

Spontaneous abortion. *See* Miscarriage.

Sports injuries. Health problems caused by sports activities. All sports injuries should be examined by a doctor. Rest, followed by exercise of the injured arm, leg, or other affected body part, is commonly prescribed. The specific sport that caused the damage may need to be stopped for a time, to allow the injured part to heal and regain strength.

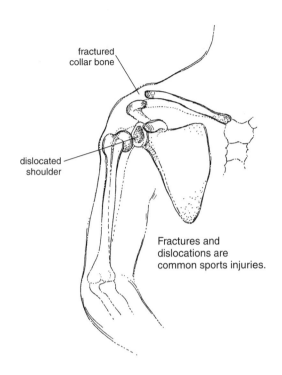

fractured collar bone

dislocated shoulder

Fractures and dislocations are common sports injuries.

Common Sports Injuries

Pulled muscle, strain, tear. If too much stress is placed on a muscle, some muscle fibers may be damaged or tear, causing pain and swelling. The hamstring muscle on the back of the thigh is a common area for this kind of injury.

Sprain. A sprain is an injury to the ligaments, the connective tissue that holds bones and joints in place. Too much stress can stretch or tear a ligament, causing pain, swelling of the joint, and discoloration. Sprains often occur in the ankles and knees.

Dislocation. A forceful blow or injury may cause a dislocation in a joint; the end of a bone is pulled out of the joint. Swelling, inability to move the joint, pain, and discoloration are signs of a dislocation. Dislocations most often occur in shoulder joints, knees, and fingers.

Fracture. A fracture or break may occur when too much stress or pressure is put on a bone. In a closed fracture, the bone is broken, but it does not stick out of the skin. In an open fracture, the broken bone is visible, protruding through the skin.

Stress fracture. Repeated or prolonged stress on a bone can cause a hairline crack, a stress fracture, in the bone. There is pain at the point of the break. Stress fractures are most common in the foot bones and in the tibia, or shinbone, but can occur anywhere.

Shin splints. Pain in the front part of the leg, below the knee, is often described as shin splints. The cause of the pain may be a muscle tear, a stress fracture, or inflammation of the membrane covering the shin bones.

Hand injuries. Finger, hand, and wrist bones can be broken or dislocated and tendons can be damaged through impact, overuse, or overstretching.

Head injuries. A hard impact can cause a skull fracture or damage to the brain. Symptoms include headache, dizziness, bleeding, and loss of consciousness. Head injuries require emergency medical attention.

Knee injuries. A forceful impact, sudden strain, or repeated stress on the knee may damage the ligaments, bones, or cartilage causing pain, a grinding or popping sensation in the knee, or swelling.

Spotting between periods. Small amounts of blood-tinged vaginal discharge. Spotting is usually of no significance when it occurs at the beginning of a period or at the start of labor in a woman who is about to give birth.

Spotting at other times may indicate a hormonal imbalance or abnormality in the female organs. In a pregnant woman spotting may indicate a problem with the pregnancy. Frequent spotting (except at the beginning of a regular period) should be investigated by a physician, and treatment started for any abnormal condition.

Sprain. Partial or complete tear of a ligament, the strong, fiberlike tissue that connects bones. A sprain may occur during a sports activity and may cause pain and swelling.

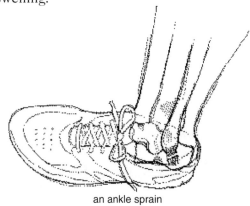
an ankle sprain

Rest, an ice pack, elevation of the affected part, and a pain reliever such as aspirin or ibuprofen will reduce pain and start the healing process. Depending on the severity of the sprain, healing may take from a few days to several weeks.

Sputum. Mucous material from the nose, throat, windpipe (trachea), or lungs that collects in the mouth. People who have a respiratory infection often produce increased amounts of sputum when they cough or clear the throat. Thick or discolored (gray, green, yellow) sputum may indicate a bacterial infection.

Squint. *See* Eye disorders, strabismus.

Stages of development. *See* Tanner stages.

Staining. *See* Spotting.

Staphylococcus (Staph). A common type of bacteria that can cause many different infections. These range from a pimple or boil to dangerous, sometimes life-threatening infections that involve one or more organs or spread through the bloodstream.

Starvation, compulsive. An eating disorder. *See* Anorexia nervosa.

Statutory rape. Sexual intercourse by an adult with a minor is considered rape even if the minor consents. Rape of any kind is a crime punishable by law. Legally there are several degrees of statutory rape:
- Statutory rape, first degree: sexual intercourse of a man age eighteen or over with a girl less than eleven years of age
- Statutory rape, second degree: sexual intercourse of a man age eighteen or over with a female age fourteen or under
- Statutory rape, third degree: sexual intercourse of a man age twenty-one or older with a female less than seventeen years of age

STD. *See* Sexually transmitted disease.

STD hotline. A telephone service providing confidential, accurate information about sexually transmitted diseases. *See* Appendix A: Hotlines.

Sterilization (reproductive). A surgical procedure that makes it impossible to have a child.

In male sterilization, surgery (vasectomy) is performed to cut and tie the tubes (vas deferens) that carry sperm from the testicles. After the surgery, no sperm are present in the ejaculate, making pregnancy impossible.

In female sterilization, surgery (tubal ligation) is performed to "tie the woman's tubes"—that is, to close the fallopian tubes. As a result, eggs can no longer meet sperm to be fertilized or travel to the uterus and start a pregnancy.

Steroids. Synthetic drugs similar to the hormones produced by the pituitary and the adrenal glands. Steroid drugs are used to treat a variety of diseases, including asthma and eczema.

Some athletes illegally use one class of steroids, anabolic steroids, to build muscle

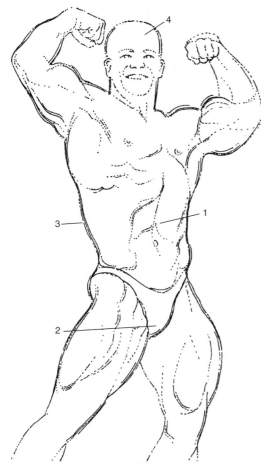

While anabolic steroids may build muscle mass, they may also lead to:

1. liver cancer
2. atrophied testicles
3. stunted growth
4. psychological instability, violence

mass and overall strength to improve their athletic performance. This practice is dangerous as well as illegal. Used for any length of time, anabolic steroids cause major physical and mental problems. In the short run, these drugs may improve physical performance; but if used over longer periods, harmful physical and mental changes develop. These include:

Physical changes: in teenagers, little or no further growth, increase of blood pressure, decrease of male sex hormone levels, liver damage, infertility, and (in boys) possible enlargement of the breasts.

Mental changes: irritability, aggressive behavior, suspiciousness, and violence.

Stethoscope. A medical instrument used to listen to the sounds of the heart, large blood vessels, and some other organs. This process is called auscultation. The stethoscope permits external examination of some of the heart's functions, and of other body areas, to detect signs of abnormality.

The stethoscope consists of two earpieces, attached to plastic or rubber tubing. The tubing ends in a cone, which is placed on the chest or other part of the body to be examined.

Stinger (burner). An injury sustained during a head-on tackle. The impact causes shock waves along the spinal cord, back, and arms, causing a numb or burning sensation for a while.

A person who has had a stinger must be examined by a doctor before resuming any sports activities. This is needed to rule out any unrecognized congenital conditions (abnormalities existing since birth) of the cervical (neck) bones that surround the spinal column. Specific treatment is needed if such a problem is diagnosed.

Stomachache. Achy, burning discomfort in the stomach area. It may be caused by irritating foods, overeating, infection, tension, stress, or an ulcer. A mild stomachache usually disappears if you rest, eat bland, non-greasy foods (tea, toast), avoid stress and tension, and refrain from taking over-the-counter drugs such as Pepto-Bismol, Maalox, or Tums until after a medical checkup.

If you have a severe stomachache with persistent cramps, diarrhea, or vomiting for more than several hours, see your doctor or go to a hospital emergency room. These symptoms may be signs of an acute illness that requires prompt medical attention.

Stomach ulcer. Irritation, inflammation, and breakdown of an area in the stomach wall, caused by excessive acid secretion which has destroyed part of the stomach lining. Acid overload may be caused by stress, tension, anxiety, drugs, alcohol, and smoking.

An ulcer may appear at any age. People who are perfectionists, who diet excessively, or who have experienced some form of trauma often develop an ulcer. *See also* Stress; Ulcer.

Recent research indicates that bacteria called *Helicobacter pylori (H.pylori)* may be involved in the development of ulcers of the stomach and duodenum (the first segment of the small intestine). Antibiotics and other medications are used to eliminate the bacteria, and allow for the healing of the ulcer.

Ulcer symptoms include a burning sensation in the stomach, which may spread through the chest (heartburn). A medical examination is needed to confirm the diagnosis and reveal the location of the ulcer.

Treatment depends on the location, size, and severity of the ulcer. Early diagnosis and prompt medication will stop attacks of pain, start the healing process, and prevent further ulcer development. The following measures can relieve pain and promote healing:
- Eat frequent small meals
- Use antacid medication such as Maalox,

Gelusil, or a stronger prescribed medicine
- Try to get adequate rest, avoid tension, anxiety, and stress
- Seek out counseling or other treatment for personal problems that may have contributed to the development of the ulcer.

Stone ache. *See* Blue balls.

Strabismus. *See* Eye disorders.

Strain, muscle. Muscle discomfort or pain following excessive stretching or tearing of a muscle or its attached tendon.

Strains occur in three degrees of severity:
- Strain, first degree: a slight tear with minimal loss of function
- Strain, second degree: a moderate tear with some loss of function
- Strain, third degree: a severe tear with nearly complete loss of function

A mild strain (first degree) is treated with Rest, Ice, Compression, and Elevation (RICE) until swelling and pain have decreased and function has returned. Second- and third-degree strains need to be checked and treated by a physician.

Street drugs. Drugs not obtained in drug stores, but available from dealers who sell drugs on the street. Many street drugs are illegal drugs, used mainly by people who abuse or sell these drugs, most of which are harmful to the body. The actual chemical contents of the drugs often vary from one batch to the next, with more or less of a given drug in any pill or capsule. The material may also be contaminated by dirt and other substances. *See* Appendix C: Street Drugs.

Streptococcus (Strep). A type of bacteria that may cause a variety of serious infections, including strep throat. Strep infections need to be treated with antibiotics.

Stress. A mental state that may develop when a person is under great pressure. Fam-

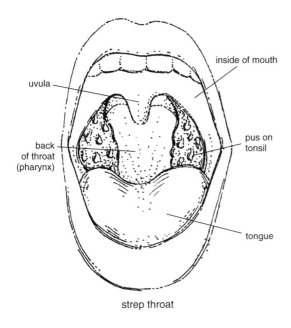

uvula

inside of mouth

back
of throat
(pharynx)

pus on
tonsil

tongue

strep throat

ily problems, financial difficulties, problems at school or in a relationship, and illness or death in the family may all produce stress. Stress can lead to mental and physical symptoms that may become overwhelming if they are not recognized and dealt with.

Mental symptoms of stress include:

- Depression
- Loss of interest in various activities
- Nervousness
- Short temper
  Physical symptoms of stress include:
- Headache
- Stomachache
- Loss of appetite
- Overeating
- Fatigue

The best way to overcome stress is to search for its causes and try to eliminate them. A counselor can help to find out the underlying causes. If the problem cannot be solved quickly, the counselor can suggest methods that will help solve it and reduce stress over a period of time. Discussing the stressful problem often provides relief.

Stress fracture. Tiny breaks, usually of the shinbone, caused by physical stress and trauma. Stress fractures often fail to heal because the stress and trauma are repeated.

Symptoms include pain, tenderness, and limping. Ordinary X rays may not reveal the problem. Special procedures such as a bone scan may be needed to make the correct diagnosis.

Stress fracture may occur in the long bones of the foot in athletes who put a lot of strain on the tips of these bones while running, and during other sports. Symptoms include pain in the involved area. Treatment includes rest, cessation of sports involving the painful area, and changing to a sport that exerts less stress on the legs and feet. Good quality running or other sports shoes are essential for prevention, and as treatment. Exercises and gradual resumption of the sport are also part of the treatment.

Preventive measures: Warm up (a few minutes of slow, relaxed exercising) before starting sports activities; careful stretching of leg muscles prior to starting sports activities; and cooling down (gradual slowdown rather than a sudden stop of sports activity) help to avoid stress fractures.

Stretch marks (striae). Marks that develop on the abdomen, thighs, and other areas caused a period of rapid physical growth and development. Stretch marks often occur in obese persons, pregnant women, and sometimes in teens. The marks fade over time but may not disappear. They are not necessarily a sign of poor health.

Stutter. *See* Speech defect.

Stye. *See* Eye disorders.

Subcutaneous (sc). Located under the skin. A subcutaneous injection, for example, is given under the skin.

Subluxation. Partial or complete dislocation of a bone or joint. May be congenital or caused by trauma. Treatment depends on the affected bone or joint and may involve the use of a cast or other measures prescribed by an orthopedic surgeon.

Substance abuse. *See* Drug abuse.

Suction lipectomy. *See* Liposuction.

Sudden infant death syndrome (SIDS). The sudden unexpected death of an apparently healthy baby or very young child due to unknown causes. Research is continuing to learn the cause of death in these babies. Some researchers believe that an unrecognized respiratory ailment is responsible. Others suspect a number of other causes, such as passive smoke inhalation, sleeping on the stomach, and natural fiber mattresses.

Suicide. Taking one's own life. Some people become so depressed that life seems too painful or no longer worth living. Young people may feel this way if they are failing in school, have major problems with parents, lack friends, or experience the breakup of a relationship or the death of a family member or friend.

Immediate help is needed for anyone

Warning signs of suicide

- Severe depression, with loss of appetite, troubled sleep patterns, loss of interest in life, and feelings of despair.
- Withdrawal. Loss of interest in friends and activities. Isolation.
- Severe mood swings.
- Changes in behavior and personality.
- Threats of suicide.
- Dangerous risk-taking, disregard of personal safety.
- Heavy use of alcohol or drugs.
- Giving away valued possessions.
- A crisis. A death of a friend or family member, parents' divorce, the end of a relationship, a severe disappointment.
- Frequent talk of death and dying.

If you are concerned about a friend's behavior, talk to a teacher, counselor, doctor, or other adult.

---

who expresses a wish to die. Counseling, medication to overcome the depression, and hospitalization may save the life of someone who is too depressed to want to live, and further treatment may help him or her to overcome suicidal feelings and enjoy life.

Sunburn. The result of exposure to sunlight. Too much exposure may cause the skin to burn, raising blisters and causing other damage. Exposure to sun over time can lead to skin cancer. Sunburn can be prevented by covering body areas with clothing, using sunscreen, and avoiding frequent, long exposure to sunlight. Winter sunlight, especially when reflecting off snow, can also cause sunburn. *See also* Sunscreen.

Sunscreen. A preparation that blocks the sun's rays and prevents burning of the skin when exposed to sunlight. A pigment called melanin protects skin against sunburn, but the amount of melanin varies in different people. Those who are light-skinned and fair-complexioned have almost no melanin and are at great risk of sunburn. Those with darker complexions have more of the pigment but still need protection against strong sunlight.

Good sunscreens are available as lotions or creams. They come in several strengths and either block the sun's ultraviolet rays, or contain protective chemical agents such as para-aminobenzoic acid. If you are fair-skinned and expect to be exposed to sun, use a sunscreen with maximum protection. The protective capacity is designated on the container by the SPF (sun protection factor) number. Use a protection factor of 15 to 33 if your complexion is fair, and a protection factor of 8 to 15 if your complexion is medium or dark.

Choose a sunscreen labeled "broad spectrum protection" to protect yourself from all of the sun's rays. To keep your skin soft, apply a moisturizer after washing off the sunscreen. Remember, the sun dries as well as burns your skin. If you have sensitive lips, buy a lipstick or a protective cream (Chapstick, Blistex) that contains sunscreen protection.

Sunstroke. A dangerous condition that may develop if you are active and exposed to hot sun for a long time—during a ball game, for example. Sunstroke occurs when the body cannot get rid of stored-up heat. Symptoms include high body temperature (up to 106°F.), absence of sweating, dry skin, dehydration, headache, numbness, rapid pulse and breathing, confusion, and coma, which may end in death if treatment is not started immediately. For emergency treatment, *see* First Aid section.

Emergency sunstroke treatment includes:
- Immediate removal of the victim from the sun into a cool area
- Hospitalization
- Immersion in a tub of cool water or placement on an ice-cooled mattress (hypothermia mattress)
- Infusion of cool intravenous liquids to replenish essential body fluids

Take the following special precautions against sunstroke:
- Don't overexercise when it is very hot
- Drink plenty of cool fluids
- Get out of the sun to a cool place at frequent intervals

Suppository. A small, cone-shaped tablet containing medication. A suppository is inserted into the rectum to treat such problems as itching or hemorrhoids. Suppositories are inserted into the vagina to treat inflammation or infection. Suppositories may also be used when a person is suffering from nausea and can't keep down medicine taken by mouth.

Surgery, breast reduction. *See* Breast reduction.

Surgery, plastic. *See* Plastic surgery.

Surgery, reconstructive. *See* Plastic surgery.

Swimmer's ear. An infectious condition that develops when a person's ears are exposed to water for long periods—for example, while swimming. Symptoms include itching, pain, drainage, and possible hearing loss. The changes in the skin of the inner ear may also predispose a person to the development of ear infection. Consult a doctor if you have any of these symptoms. Prescribed ear medication clears up swimmer's ear.

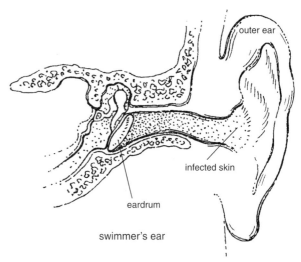

swimmer's ear

If you are a frequent swimmer, you may prevent swimmer's ear by taking these precautions: (1) wear a tight-fitting bathing cap; (2) ask your doctor for a prescription for alcohol-based eardrops, and (3) keep your ears clean and dry at all times.

Swollen glands. Enlarged glands in one or several parts of the body that may signal an infection or other illness. Swollen glands in the neck may indicate an infection in the head, face, neck, or throat. Enlarged glands in the groin may indicate an infection in the lower abdomen or genital tract. In some people, enlarged glands are a sign of a growth or a blood disease.

If you have swollen glands, consult your doctor or school health clinic. You need a prompt examination and treatment if an infection or other illness is found.

Symptoms. Physical or mental changes that indicate a developing or full-blown mental or physical illness.

Symptoms help to make the diagnosis. Physicians and other health professionals learn to recognize symptoms and groups of symptoms. They can tell the symptoms of one illness from those of a similar illness, which helps them to make the correct diagnosis.

For example, if a person complains of abdominal pain, the doctor takes a health and family history by asking questions about recent and earlier illnesses, and about family members' health problems. He or she performs a physical exam and one or more tests, then evaluates the findings and makes the diagnosis. The vague complaint of abdominal pain can now be identified as indigestion, intestinal flu, an infection, an ulcer, or a serious illness such as cancer. To make an accurate diagnosis of other illnesses, further tests may be necessary.

The process of diagnosing mental illness is similar to that used in diagnosing a physical illness. A careful examination uncovers the information the doctor needs to decide the nature and probable cause of mental symptoms. The symptoms may include excessive sadness, unwarranted excitement, or behavioral changes in which a normally peaceful person becomes aggressive, violent, or withdrawn.

Since mental symptoms can also be signs of a physical illness, a physical examination may be performed to make the correct diagnosis.

Syndrome. A group of illnesses or health problems that appear at the same time and result from the same cause. AIDS is a syndrome because it consists of a number of health problems that often appear at the same time. All are caused by HIV infection.

Syphilis (lues). A sexually transmitted disease. Syphilis is a progressive disease that gradually affects the entire body if it is not treated. Syphilis occurs in several stages: primary, secondary, latent, and tertiary.

Cause: Syphilis is caused by the spirochete *Treponema pallidum*, a bacterium.

Primary syphilis begins with a chancre (small lesion) on the penis or vagina. A chancre may also occur on the lips, tongue, or tonsils.

The chancre appears from nine to ninety days after discharge from an infected sexual partner's lesion is rubbed into the healthy partner's skin. The chancre is usually painless, but may be felt as a lump in the tonsillar area, usually on the left tonsil.

Secondary syphilis starts from nine to ninety days after the appearance of the chancre if the first stage has not been treated. Symptoms include flulike feelings—headache, fever, sore throat, runny nose, tearing, and joint pain. Also commonly found: weight loss, enlarged glands throughout the body, and a rash on the trunk, shoulders, and arms. Later, a different type of rash develops on the face and trunk, in the mouth, and in the moist areas of the genitals. The rash usually does not itch. The central nervous system (brain, spinal cord, nerves) may become involved during this stage.

Latent syphilis usually begins a year or more after the initial infection if no treatment has been given. This stage may last for a few years or for the rest of an untreated person's life. Symptoms include recurrences of the infectious rash. After some years, an untreated person may develop tertiary syphilis.

Tertiary (late) syphilis develops as the last stage in untreated persons, three to ten years after the initial infection. Painful lumps, called gumma, appear in various body areas. The heart may become involved. The brain and spinal cord nerves may be affected, leading to confusion, seizures, weakness, and difficulty in walking, along with other serious problems. Fortunately, tertiary syphilis is rare in this country because antibiotic treatment is usually given early in the disease, preventing this deadly late stage.

The most important thing to remember about syphilis is this: If you notice symptoms of a chancre on the genitals or lips, or inside the mouth, go to a doctor or health service immediately. A blood test (VDRL or rapid plasma reagin test, RPR) will show if you have syphilis. If you do, effective antibiotic treatment will quickly cure the disease.

Syphilis, congenital. Syphilis transmitted by an infected pregnant woman to the fetus. Symptoms in a newborn baby include a rash or small blisters on the palms and soles, nose and mouth, and in the diaper area.

Blood-tinged or pus-filled nasal discharge, enlarged lymph glands in various body areas, and other abnormal conditions may develop and the infection may affect the liver, brain, and nervous system. Babies with syphilis often do not thrive like normal babies. They look like little old men. Effective treatment is available for babies. However, treatment of the pregnant woman will prevent congenital syphilis in her children.

Systemic lupus erythematosus (SLE). A chronic disease of unknown cause that involves the autoimmune system. SLE occurs primarily in young women and occasionally in children. Symptoms of SLE include inflammation or infection of connective and other tissues. Many different organs may be affected, such as the lungs, heart, kidneys, and joints. There is no cure for this disease. Symptoms are treated as they arise. *See also* Lupus erythematosus.

T

Tampon. A device inserted into the vagina to absorb the menstrual flow. The tampon consists of a stiff tube (for easy vaginal inser-

How to insert a tampon

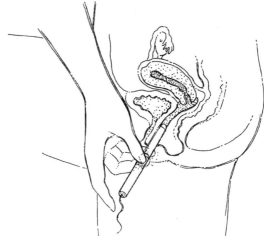

Using the stiff cover as a guide, insert the tampon into the vagina.

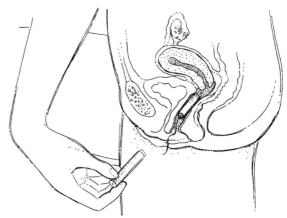

Once the tampon is securely placed in the vagina, remove the cover. The string is later used to pull out the tampon.

tion) filled with compressed cotton. After the tampon is in place, the stiff casing is removed and discarded. The cotton plug expands inside the vagina, soaking up menstrual blood. Some tampons consist of compressed cotton plugs without a casing.

Tampons should be replaced several times a day, depending on the amount of flow. When the tampon becomes saturated, it cannot absorb more menstrual secretions. Superabsorbant tampons must be replaced also, even if not saturated. If a tampon stays in the vagina for more than twenty-four hours it may cause a dangerous infection, such as toxic shock syndrome. *See also* Sanitary napkin; Toxic shock syndrome.

Tanner stages. A system of measurements designed by physician J. M. Tanner to track physical development from childhood through adolescence to adulthood. The measurements are divided into five stages:

Tanner stage 1: Applies to boys and girls ages eight to eleven. Internal signs of puberty: in girls, enlargement of the ovaries; in boys, enlargement of the testicles; in boys and girls, production of sex hormones. External signs of puberty: pubic hair not yet visible.

Tanner stage 2: Applies to girls average ages eleven to twelve, and boys ages eleven to thirteen. Signs of early puberty in girls: appearance of breast buds, some pubic hair, rapid growth. In boys: testicles and scrotum grow larger; increase in height and weight, muscle mass, and fat; pubic hair starts to grow.

Tanner stage 3: Applies to girls average ages twelve to thirteen, boys average ages thirteen to sixteen. In girls, changes include enlarging breasts, coarsening of pubic hair, and increase in vaginal size; a whitish vaginal discharge may appear; menstrual periods may begin. Changes in boys include an increase in the size of the penis, testicles, and scrotum; deepening of the voice; and beginning growth of facial hair.

Tanner stage 4: Applies to girls average ages thirteen to fourteen, boys average ages fourteen to fifteen. In girls, the pubic hair pattern becomes triangular, underarm hair starts to grow, and ovulation and menstruation begin. In boys, the testicles and scrotum continue to grow, the penis grows in width and length, the voice deepens further, underarm and facial hair continue to grow, and ejaculations may occur.

Tanner stage 5: Applies to girls average ages fourteen to sixteen, boys average ages fifteen to sixteen. In girls, it is the final growth stage of breasts and pubic hair; hormonal development is complete and the appearance is that of a young adult woman. In boys, genital, pubic, and facial hair growth are now complete, regular shaving is necessary, and chest hair may continue to grow; appearance is that of young adult male.

There is a wide age range for each Tanner stage; some girls and boys reach maturity earlier than others. This is normal, and neither early nor somewhat later maturity is a cause for concern.

Important: If a young person notices few or no signs of puberty by age sixteen, a doctor should be consulted to see if there is any cause that may require medical attention.

Tapeworm. *See* Parasite infestation.

Tattoo, body. A tattoo is a design etched into the skin with indelible ink. That means it is there to stay, and would require intervention by a skin specialist if the tattooed person decided to have it removed.

Some teens and adults believe tattoos, or "body art," are attractive. Others wish to "make a statement" of some sort—about their beliefs, their work (as a biker might have a motorcycle tattooed on the body), a club or other affiliation—or are seeking attention. To create a tattoo, a professional tattooer uses colored inks and a vibrating electric needle to imbed a chosen design at the selected location on the skin. A typical tattoo takes a half hour to an hour to complete, and the process is painful. The site is sore and is kept bandaged. After about a week, the scabs fall off and the tattoo is visible.

Caution: Inadequately sterilized needles can transmit serious infections such as hepatitis, bacterial or other infections, or even the AIDS virus. Allergic reactions to the tattoo inks may develop in some people. Tattoo removal requires laser treatment or another type of surgical process, and usually results in a mark or scar. A safer alternative to tattoos is body decoration by the use of transfer decals or makeup pencils. These can be self-applied, and removed when no longer wanted, with no health hazards.

TB. *See* Tuberculosis.

T cells. A class of white blood cells called lymphocytes that help the body to fight infection. People with advanced HIV infection and those with AIDS have too few T cells to fight infection. This condition allows germs to invade the body and cause serious, often life-threatening, infections. *See also* Lymphocytes.

Teeth. Teeth are essential in chewing food, and in forming speech sounds, and give shape to the face *See also* Dental care; Dental caries.

Temperature (body). The degree of heat in the body. In humans, the average body temperature is 98.6°F (37.8°C), but some people have a somewhat lower or higher normal body temperature. Body temperature varies during the day, going up somewhat in the afternoon, and dropping during the night.

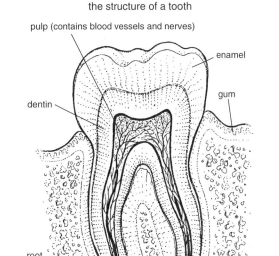

the structure of a tooth

pulp (contains blood vessels and nerves)

enamel

gum

dentin

root canals

bone

It also fluctuates with activity, and with the environment.

Illness may produce a rise in temperature (fever) while other conditions may lower it. A moderate or high fever requires medical care, as does an abnormally low temperature. Body temperature is measured with oral, rectal, or underarm thermometers, or with an electronic thermometer. Follow the instructions provided with the thermometer.

The body has different methods to regulate its temperature, to keep it fairly constant in normal circumstances. The hypothalamus (in the brain), for example, acts as a thermostat to regulate temperature. So do the blood and the sweat glands. *See also* Blood.

Tendinitis. Inflammation of a tendon, the fibrous tissue that connects muscle to bone. Irritated or inflamed tendons cause pain or tenderness.

Rest, application of ice, and anti-inflammatory medications such as aspirin or Advil will relieve tendinitis. After the pain disappears, use stretching and warm-up exercises to get ready to resume physical activities. *See also* Patellar tendinitis.

Tendon. Tough, fibrous tissue that connects muscle to bone. The Achilles tendon, for example, connects the calf muscles to the heel bone.

Tennis elbow. Irritation or inflammation of the elbow caused by overuse or improper technique in sports. Tennis elbow is a form of tendinitis. *See also* Tendinitis.

Tension headache. A head pain that appears when a person is subjected to stress or tension. Stress causes the muscles of the neck and shoulders to tighten and contract, causing the pain. Aspirin or another pain reliever will ease the headache, but the cause of stress must be found and eliminated or the headache may recur.

Teratogen. Any chemical, drug, or other substance which, if taken by a pregnant woman, may cause an abnormality or deformity in the fetus. Teratogenic substances include alcohol, certain antibiotics, anticancer drugs, and some pain relievers.

Termination of pregnancy. *See* Abortion.

Testicle. One of the two oval-shaped organs located inside the scrotum. The testicles produce the male hormone testosterone, as well as sperm. (Slang for testicles: balls, jewels, nuts). *See also* Reproductive system, male.

Testicle, floating. A testicle that may rise into the lower part of the abdomen because it is not firmly attached to the wall of the scrotum. While in the lower abdomen, a floating testicle may seem to have disappeared. Gentle pressure can usually return it to the scrotum.

Testicle, undescended. A testicle located in the lower abdomen instead of the scrotum, where it belongs. Normally, both testicles descend (move down) from the lower abdomen, where they develop in the fetus, to the scrotum by the time the baby is born. In some cases, a newborn boy's testicle (one or both) remains in the abdomen instead of descending to the scrotum. This condition should be corrected during the first year of life, either with medication or surgery. If it is not, the testicle may become damaged beyond repair and have to be removed. In some cases, boys whose undescended testicle was not removed may develop cancer in that testicle.

Testicular cancer. An abnormal growth of cells in one or both testicles. A male who has an undescended testicle that was not removed may develop testicular cancer. Fortunately, this and other types of testicular cancer can be cured, if detected and treated at an early stage. *See also* Testicular self-examination.

Testicular self-examination. A simple procedure to detect unusual lumps or bumps on the testicles. Every young man should perform a weekly testicular self-exam, easily done while taking a shower or bath:

1. Place one testicle between your thumb and fingers.

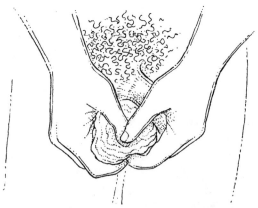

In a testicular self-examination, feel for any lumps (about the size of a pea) on the front or side of the testicle.

2. Gently roll the testicle around several times. Its surface should feel smooth and non-tender.
3. If you feel or see anything unusual, contact your doctor immediately for an examination.

Testicular torsion. A surgical emergency that occurs when a free-floating testicle becomes twisted on its cord and in the veins and arteries that nurture it. There may be no known cause, or it may occur after strenuous exercise, or as a result of faulty development before birth. Severe pain, nausea, and vomiting, followed by fever and swelling, are the symptoms. The blood vessel tangle must be surgically unraveled within a few hours, or the testicle will die and require surgical removal.

Testosterone. The male sex hormone produced in the testicles. During puberty, testosterone causes the development of body hair and the deepening of the voice.

Tetanus (lockjaw). A dangerous, frequently fatal infection caused by the tetanus germ, which enters through a cut or puncture of the skin. This may happen when a person steps on a nail while barefoot, or is cut by a rusty knife or by broken glass.

Without treatment, the infected person develops severe muscle spasms (the jaw may lock, hence "lockjaw") and seizures. Death often follows. Anyone who receives a "dirty" injury should immediately go to a hospital emergency room and receive specific treatment (tetanus immunoglobulin, human, and antibiotics) to prevent tetanus infection.

Tetanus toxoid is a vaccine that provides immunity against the infection. After age fourteen, a booster injection of tetanus toxoid given every ten years will maintain immunity. *See also* Immunization.

Tetanus booster shot. A repeat injection of tetanus toxoid to maintain immunity against tetanus infection.

Tetanus immune globulin, human. A medication given to a person who receives a "dirty" wound, as when the skin is cut by glass or punctured by a nail, allowing tetanus germs to enter the bloodstream. *See also* Tetanus.

Tetanus toxoid. A vaccine given to immunize people against tetanus infection. *See also* Tetanus.

Thalassemia. An inherited blood disease that affects the normal development of hemoglobin and red blood cells. A person with thalassemia has unusually small red blood cells that have a very short life span. Other symptoms include anemia, an enlarged spleen, and a poorly developed body.

A person who inherits a thalassemia gene from one parent usually has a mild form of the disease; with thalassemia genes inherited from both parents, severe disease is likely.

Thelarche. Development of the breasts during puberty.

Thrombocytopenia (thrombocytopenic purpura, TP). A disease of reduced platelets, a blood component that helps clotting of the blood after a cut, injury, or surgery. The cause may be unknown, a viral infection, or certain medications. With poor clotting, skin bruises easily when touched, or gums may bleed freely when brushed. Hormonal drugs such as steroids help to stabilize this disease.

Thrush. A fungus infection that causes patches of white material to appear on the tongue and elsewhere in an infected person's mouth. Healthy babies or children sometimes develop thrush. People who have damaged immune systems, such as those with AIDS, commonly have this disease. The treatment is antifungal medication.

Thyroid. A gland located in the midsection of the neck, which regulates many different body functions. The thyroid acts as an accelerator and as a brake. When the gland is overactive (secretes more than normal amounts of thyroid hormone), a person feels as if he or she is running a race, even while standing still. The heart beats rapidly, and blood pressure may be elevated. When the thyroid is less active (secretes less than normal amounts of thyroid hormone), a person may feel as if he or she is living in slow motion.

Blood tests are used to monitor thyroid function, and to detect any problems. In most cases, abnormal thyroid function can be corrected with medication, but surgery is sometimes necessary.

Thyroid function tests (TFTs). Tests to determine the blood level of thyroid hormone. The results show if a patient has low, normal, or high levels of the hormone. Treatment is given if the levels are too high or too low for normal functioning.

Thyroid-stimulating hormone (TSH). A hormone produced in the brain that regulates thyroid function.

Ticks. *See* Lyme disease; Appendix F: First Aid, tick bites.

Tinea corporis. *See* Ringworm.

Tinea cruris. *See* Jock itch.

Tinea versicolor. A skin infection caused by the fungus *Pityrosporum orbiculare*. White, tan, or brown lesions appear on the chest, neck or face. It is commonly seen in older adolescents and young adults. Treatment consists of a variety of prescribed medications. Normal skin color returns on exposure to sunlight.

Tonsillitis. Infection of the tonsils, the two glands located behind the tongue at the back of the throat. Tonsillitis is often caused by a simple flu virus. Symptoms include a scratchy sore throat, a raspy voice, and a slight fever.

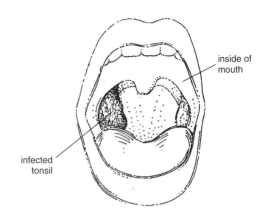

inside of mouth

infected tonsil

Tonsillitis may also be caused by bacteria (streptococcus, gonococcus) or by a virus (herpes virus, Epstein-Barr virus). With these organisms as the cause, the affected person may feel more ill. White patches may appear in the throat in these severe cases of infection.

Bacterial tonsillitis can be cured quickly with antibiotics, but there is no effective medication for the viral infections. Rest, fluids, and pain medicines such as Tylenol, provide relief.

Torn ligament. *See* Ligament, torn.

Torticollis. Stiffness and muscle spasms on either side of the neck, making it difficult to move the head from side to side. The causes include direct injury to the neck, overexertion, and strenuous exercise that strains the neck muscles. *See* Muscle, pulled.

Pain relievers, anti-inflammatory medication, and muscle relaxants are used for treatment. As with most muscle injuries, ice is helpful when used during the first twenty-four to forty-eight hours, followed by the application of heat. In moderate to severe cases, a cervical collar (neck brace) can reduce muscle tension and discomfort.

Toxic shock syndrome (TSS). A serious, sometimes fatal infection caused by the staphylococcus organism. This infection occurs mainly after the use of superabsorbent menstrual tampons, especially if they are not changed every three to four hours. Symptoms include a high fever, chills, weakness, a rash on the hands and feet, and severe diarrhea.

To prevent TSS: (1) wash your hands before inserting a tampon; (2) do not use superabsorbent tampons; (3) change tampons every three to four hours during the day, even when the menstrual flow is light.

Toxoplasmosis. An infection caused by the parasite *Toxoplasma gondii*. In most people, this infection is not usually serious. It is dangerous for pregnant women, however, because it can cause a miscarriage, a premature birth, or major illness in the newborn baby. In people with AIDS, the infection may travel to the brain and start a deadly abscess.

The toxo germ is often found in homes with cats. It is therefore important to wash your hands after handling a cat or cleaning a litter box.

Tranquilizer (downer). A drug that relieves tension, anxiety, and nervousness. *See* Appendix B, Anti-anxiety drugs.

Transfusion (blood). Administration of a quantity of blood, usually a pint at a time, to a person who has lost blood due to injury, surgery, or an illness that decreases production of blood or its components. A person may receive a transfusion of whole blood or only the component needed. Someone with a low platelet count, for example, may receive a platelet transfusion.

In the United States, donor blood is checked to make sure it contains no infectious organisms, ensuring a high degree of safety. Both the donor blood and the recipient are also tested for blood type and compatibility, to make sure the donor blood matches that of the recipient.

Transgender. *See* Transsexual.

Transsexual. A man or woman who wants a sex change. Male or female transsexuals may undergo hormone therapy and eventually surgery to change their sex organs and general appearance to that of a person of the opposite sex.

Before any surgical procedures (removal of the genital organs in men, or creation of a penis in women) are performed, the female transsexual takes male hormone therapy and the male transsexual takes female hormone therapy for one or more years. At the end of that time, and after psychiatric evaluation, the sex change surgery may be performed.

Transvestite. A person who enjoys and feels comfortable dressed in clothing of the opposite sex, without wishing to change his or her sex.

Trauma. Serious physical, mental, or emotional injury.

Traveling out of the country

If you plan to travel, work, or study outside the country, follow the guidelines below to protect your health. Water supplies and sanitation standards may not be fully safe in some developing countries.

Before you go

1. About two months (or earlier) before you leave, check with your doctor, local public health office, the embassy of the country you plan to visit, or the U.S. Center for Disease Control and Prevention in Atlanta, Georgia, to find out about any current health problems or epidemics in that country, and whether any specific vaccinations are recommended or required for entry into the country.

2. At least a month before you leave, ask your doctor or local public health office when and where you can get the vaccinations you need. Some vaccines may have to be ordered for you; and you may need to start some preventive drug treatments (such as antimalaria drugs) a few weeks before you travel.

3. In the last weeks before you leave, fill prescriptions for any medications you need to take with you. Take along a copy of the prescriptions, and a copy of any prescriptions for glasses.

4. If you are going to a tropical area, take sunscreen, insect repellent, mosquito netting if you will be camping, and protective clothing.

Trench mouth. Infection of the gums caused by poor dental and mouth hygiene. The gums may turn black and bleed easily. A person with trench mouth often has an unpleasant mouth odor. Treatment includes careful cleaning of gums and teeth with a soft toothbrush. Gargling with warm saltwater (1/4 teaspoon in 1/2 glass of water) is helpful. Antibiotic medication may be prescribed. A pain reliever such as Tylenol provides comfort. A nourishing diet and plenty of fluids are essential. Smoking and spicy foods should be avoided as they irritate injured gum tissues and prevent healing.

Trichinosis. A serious parasitic infestation that may occur if a person eats uncooked or improperly cooked or processed pork that is infected by a roundworm, *Trichinella spiralis*. The larvae (immature form) of the roundworm, once inside the body, cause symptoms that include fever, abdominal pain, and diarrhea. In severe instances, there may be muscle pain and the heart and other organs may be affected.

A drug, thiabendazole, is effective, but only if taken early in the disease. The most important precaution: Never eat raw or undercooked pork, sausages, or bacon.

Trichomonas. A parasite (microscopic organism) that causes trichomoniasis. *See* Trichomoniasis.

Trichomoniasis. Infection caused by the Trichomonas organism, which mainly affects the genital organs.

Symptoms: In men, no apparent symptoms in most cases. Some women have no apparent symptoms. Other women complain of a foul, itchy, greenish-yellow vaginal discharge, soreness in the genital area, and pain while urinating.

Transmission: During sexual contact, or, rarely, by warm, moist objects (bath water, towels) used by an infected person.

Treatment: Metronidazole (Flagyl), a drug that acts specifically against protozoan organisms such as Trichomonas.

Special precautions: No sex until the infection is cleared up.

Trick knee. An unstable knee that buckles, or gives out, during certain movements. Trick knee may be caused by a partial or complete tear of a supporting ligament. *See also* Locking knee.

Trimester. A period of three months. Pregnancy generally lasts three trimesters (nine months).

Triphasic birth control pill. *See* Birth control pill.

TSS. *See* Toxic shock syndrome.

Tubal ligation. *See* Sterilization.

Tubal pregnancy (ectopic pregnancy). Implantation and development of a fertilized egg in one of the fallopian tubes instead of in the uterus.

Normally a fertilized egg travels through one of the fallopian tubes and on to the uterus where it settles and develops. However, if a female has had an infection or some other problem in the genital tract that caused

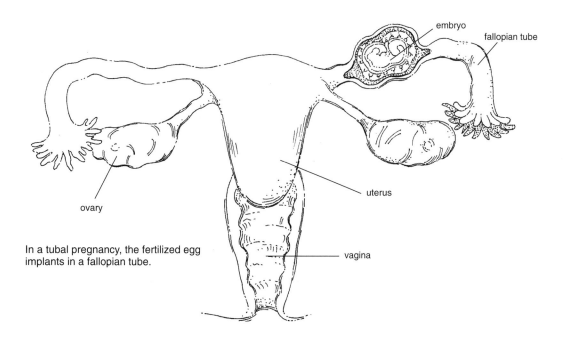

embryo

fallopian tube

uterus

vagina

ovary

In a tubal pregnancy, the fertilized egg implants in a fallopian tube.

scars and deformities of the fallopian tubes, the egg's passage may be difficult or impossible. The egg may get stuck in one of the tubes, settle in the wall, and start a pregnancy.

Tubal or ectopic pregnancy is a dangerous condition. The walls of the fallopian tubes are very thin and do not expand easily. They may burst as the fetus grows, causing a life-threatening emergency. If discovered early, medical treatment may be possible. At a later stage, surgery must be performed quickly to save the woman's life.

Tuberculosis (TB). An infectious disease that can strike people at any age.

Cause: *Mycobacterium tuberculosis*, an organism that mainly affects the lungs.

Transmission: Coughing or spitting up mucus, which spills the organisms into the air. When inhaled by others, the infection travels through their breathing passages and may infect their lungs.

Tuberculosis is diagnosed by a skin test and chest X rays. A positive skin test and a negative chest X ray indicate exposure to TB, but no active disease. A positive skin test *and* a positive chest X ray confirm active tuberculosis.

Symptoms: There may be no symptoms in the early stages of infection. After some time, the infected person complains of weight loss, fatigue, weakness, and cough, caused by bits of damaged lung tissue in the breathing passages. As the disease progresses, additional symptoms arise: fever, breathing difficulties, and chest pain.

Treatment: A person with active TB may receive one or more antibiotics that must be taken for at least nine to twelve months to cure the disease.

A person who has been exposed to TB but does not have active TB takes medication for at least six months, to prevent the development of active disease.

Complications: The disease may spread to other parts of the body. This is especially likely if an infected person (1) is not treated, (2) does not take the medication as instructed, or (3) becomes resistant to the medication.

Special precautions: Follow these guidelines to prevent the spread of TB when a family member has the disease:

- Have all members of the infected person's family tested for TB
- Keep living quarters well ventilated; open windows frequently
- Wash dishes used by an infected person in hot, soapy water
- Sleep in a different room, away from the infected person
- Use a separate toothbrush
- Instruct the person with TB to wash hands often, especially after using tissues
- Make sure the person who has TB receives periodic checkups and is given prompt treatment in case of recurrence

Tumescence. Enlargement of the penis caused by extra flow of blood into the penile blood vessels during sexual excitement. *See also* Erection.

Tumor. An abnormal growth of cells in the body. Some tumors grow slowly, others grow quickly. As the cells grow and multiply, they compete with healthy cells for nourishment. As the tumor enlarges, it may press on healthy tissue, causing damage and destruction. Some tumors grow and remain at the same site. Others may spread (metastasize) to other parts of the body. A tumor that spreads is called a malignant tumor.

Type I diabetes. *See* Diabetes mellitus.

Type 2 diabetes. *See* Diabetes mellitus.

U

Ulcer. An area of breakdown in sore or inflamed skin or mucous membrane. An ulcer may occur somewhere inside or on the surface of the body. It is sometimes caused by an irritating substance such as excess acid produced by the body. It may also be due to poor circulation in an area such as the leg or the back. *See also* Stomach ulcer.

Ulcerative colitis. *See* Colitis, ulcerative.

Underweight. Abnormally low body weight, compared with average weight based on age, height, and body frame. Low weight may be caused by poor eating habits, intentional undereating to keep body weight low, or inability to eat adequate amounts of food due to poverty or illness. If you are losing weight, consult your doctor or someone in your school health clinic.

Some teens believe they are too fat, even though their weight is normal or low for their age, height, and size. They may suffer from anorexia, a dangerous eating disorder. *See also* Anorexia nervosa.

Undescended testicle. *See* Testicle, undescended.

Universal precautions. An infection-control method used in the hospital to prevent the spread of infection, known or unknown, from one patient to another, or to a health care worker. These precautions require health care workers to:

- Wash hands before and after working with a patient
- Use gloves prior to contact (or even possible contact) with a patient's body fluids or infected body areas
- Wear a plastic apron or gown if contact with the patient is likely to soil clothing
- Use a mask and goggles to protect the mouth, nose, and eyes if there is a possibility of splashing of body or other fluids
- Dispose of needles and syringes (after giving an injection), without breaking the needle or disassembling the injection unit, into containers specifically set up for that purpose

Unplanned pregnancy. A pregnancy that is started by accident. Accidental pregnancy most often happens when a couple have sex without using contraceptive protection. Unplanned pregnancy may also occur if a contraceptive device is used incorrectly or if the device is defective.

Since pregnancy may follow any unprotected act of intercourse, including the first one, it can be prevented only if an effective contraceptive, such as the Pill, a condom, or a diaphragm, is correctly used each time a couple has sexual intercourse.

Upper respiratory infection (URI). Infection of the nose, throat, sinuses, and other breathing passages. The common cold, caused by a virus, is an upper respiratory infection. Symptoms include a runny nose, sneezing, discomfort, and sometimes a slight fever.

Treatment includes rest, lots of fluids, an antihistamine such as Benadryl or a decongestant such as Sudafed. A high fever or persistent elevated temperature may be a sign of a bacterial infection, which requires a medical checkup, and antibiotic treatment.

Ureters. Two tubes that lead, one from each kidney, to the urinary bladder, carrying urine produced in the kidneys to the bladder.

Urethra. A tube that carries off urine from the bladder to be discharged from the body. *See illustrations* The reproductive system, female and male.

Urethritis. Inflammation of the urethra (urinary tube). Men with this condition may experience a burning sensation while urinating, often accompanied by a discharge from the penis. Women may experience burning while urinating, and may have a vaginal discharge. Nonspecific urethritis commonly occurs in people infected with Chlamydia and Trichomonas organisms. *See also* Chlamydial infection; Trichomoniasis.

Urinalysis. Laboratory examination of urine to detect signs of illness or infection somewhere in the body.

Urinary tract infection (UTI). An infection of the urinary tract, which includes all the passages through which urine passes on its way from the kidneys to the outside of the body.

Urination, pain during. Discomfort or burning sensation when urinating. The cause may be infection, irritation, or inflammation somewhere in the urinary tract or at the opening (urinary meatus) where urine is discharged from the body. Pain while urinating is often a symptom of a sexually transmitted disease, or of a bladder infection. If you have pain, see your doctor to find out the cause and get effective treatment.

Urine dipstick. A test to determine the presence of blood, protein, sugar, white blood cells, and other substances in urine.

Urine toxicology. A test to determine the presence of drugs in the urine.

Urticaria. *See* Hives.

Uterus. The womb. *See slso* Reproductive system, female.

V

Vaccination. Administration of vaccine, a substance that confers immunity to a particular infection. Most vaccines are given by injection. Polio vaccine can be taken by mouth. *See also* Immunization.

Vaccine. A solution consisting of whole or fragments of killed or weakened bacteria or viruses. Vaccines are used to protect the body against various diseases caused by harmful bacteria or viruses.

This is how a vaccine works: Exposure to tiny amounts of a particular virus or bacteria, or to their weakened (inactivated) form, stimulates the body's defense (immune) system. Over time, the body produces antibodies that give immunity to the given infection that may last for several years. *See also* Immunization.

Vacuum curettage. *See* Abortion.

Vagina. A female sex organ. *See* Reproductive system, female.

Vaginal discharge. Secretion from vaginal cells containing mucus, an odorless white semiliquid substance that lubricates and cleanses the vaginal walls. This type of discharge is normal. Medical attention is needed if the discharge
- Suddenly increases greatly in amount
- Is thick, looks yellow or green, or has a foul odor
- Causes itching of the genital area
- Is accompanied by abdominal pain

Any of these may be symptoms of a vaginal infection that requires a prompt examination and treatment.

Vaginal infection. Infection of the vagina, caused by one or more organisms. Symptoms include an abnormal vaginal discharge. Common types of vaginal infections include Gardnerella, yeast, Trichomonas, gonorrhea, and Chlamydia. *See also* entries for each of these infections.

Vaginitis. A vaginal infection that produces a vaginal discharge. Young women who have a discharge need to be examined to determine what treatment is needed, and to determine whether the sexual partner needs treatment as well.

Varicella. *See* Chicken pox.

Varicocele. A condition in which varicose (swollen, enlarged) veins develop alongside the scrotum and the spermatic cord. A varico-cele is caused by a blockage of the blood flow to the testicles. Alternative pathways are formed to allow blood to nourish the affected testicle. Varicoceles are usually discovered during a testicular self-exam, when the male finds a spongy bunch of extra blood vessels that feels like a bag of worms. *See also* Testicular self-exam.

Due to decreased blood flow, the affected testicle (usually the left) is often smaller than the other one. Sperm production may also be reduced. Depending on the shortage of blood flow, surgery (varicocelectomy) may be needed to remove the varicocele, improve blood flow, and stabilize the sperm count.

Vas deferens (spermatic cord). A tube attached to each testicle. These tubes carry sperm to the right and left seminal vesicles for storage. *See* Reproductive system, male.

Vasectomy. A surgical procedure performed to cut and tie the vas deferens as a form of male birth control. *See also* Sterilization.

VD (venereal disease). A sexually transmitted disease contracted by having sex with an infected partner. The term STD (sexually transmitted disease) is more commonly used today. *See also* Sexually transmitted disease.

VD hotline, STD hotline. A telephone number for up-to-date, confidential information about sexually transmitted diseases. *See* Appendix A: Hotlines.

VDRL test (venereal disease research laboratory test). A highly reliable blood test for syphilis, a sexually transmitted disease. *See* Syphilis.

Venereal disease. *See* VD.

Venereal warts. *See* Genital warts.

Vesicle. A fluid-filled blister on the surface of the skin.

Vibrator. A hand-held, battery-driven or electrically powered device used to soothe tender and inflamed muscles. Some vibrators are used as sexual stimulators.

Viral culture. A liquid or gel used for growing viruses in a laboratory.

Viral hepatitis. *See* Hepatitis.

Virgin. A person who has never had penile–vaginal sexual intercourse. "Secondary virginity" describes the condition of a teenager who has had sexual intercourse, but has decided to abstain from further sexual experiences until he or she is older.

Virile. Refers to a male who is physically able to reproduce; also means having "masculine characteristics."

Virus. A tiny organism that grows and multiplies in living human tissues and can cause various infections or contagious diseases. Viruses are smaller than bacteria and may be submicroscopic. They are composed of a core of genetic material (RNA or DNA), surrounded by a protein coat. There are many different types of viruses.

Vision disorders, problems. *See* Eye disorders.

Vital capacity. A measurement of the amount of air exhaled from the lungs after taking in a deep breath.

Vitamins. Ingredients present in many vegetables, fruits, and other food products that keep the body healthy and help it to function.

Although most people can get the vita-

Vitamins for your body's good health

Vitamin	Benefit	Food Sources
A retinol	keeps skin, bones, teeth healthy; essential for vision and growth	green leafy vegetables, low-fat dairy products, cantaloupe, citrus fruit
B1 thiamine	helps muscle and nervous system function, helps the body burn glucose	whole-grain enriched bread, cereals, fish, pork, peas, low-fat dairy products
B2 riboflavin	promotes healthy skin, aids in digestion	low-fat milk and cheese, green leafy vegetables, whole-grain foods, lean meats, nuts, beans
B3 niacin	aids in digestion, promotes healthy skin	lean meats, poultry, fish, beans, peas, whole-grain foods, low-fat dairy products
B6 pyridoxine	aids in hemoglobin formation, helps the body use protein; helps regulate nervous system cells	fish, poultry, beans, bananas, whole-grain cereals and breads, low-fat dairy products
B12 cobalamin	assists in red and white blood cell production, aids nervous system	lean meat, poultry, fish, yeast, low-fat milk
Folic acid folacin	assists in production of blood and body cells	green leafy vegetables, beans, mushrooms, nuts
C ascorbic acid	helps growth of body cells, aids immune system, helps the body use iron	citrus fruit, cantaloupe, strawberries, cabbage family, tomatoes, peppers
D cholecalciferol	needed for bones and teeth, health of the nervous system, and blood clotting	fortified low-fat dairy foods and cereals and breads, oily fish (salmon)
E tocopherol	helps in formation and health of red blood cells	soft margarine, oils, eggs, fish, green leafy vegetables
K	needed for blood clotting	green leafy vegetables, cabbage family, fruits, low-fat milk products

mins they need from a well-balanced, nutritious diet, vitamins are also available in the form of pills. Extra vitamins are useful in treating specific vitamin deficiencies and in certain diseases. However, taking huge doses of vitamins accomplishes little and may cause health problems. Vitamins not needed by the body are usually excreted.

Voice changes. The sometimes higher, sometimes lower, voice pitch of a teenage boy going through puberty. The pitch changes are caused by the increasing amounts of testosterone, the male sex hormone produced by the testicles. Higher testosterone levels cause the vocal cords to resonate at a lower pitch, deepening the voice. Testosterone levels vary during puberty. As they go up or down, so does the pitch of the voice.

Vomiting (emesis). Regurgitating food and digestive juices from the stomach back into the mouth, and out of the body. Vomiting may be caused by an upset stomach from contaminated food, an infection, or other intestinal problems. Diseases of the food tube (gullet, stomach, intestines) and of other internal organs (liver, pancreas) may cause vomiting. Some people vomit without any physical cause, but because they are under great stress. Other causes include certain medications and, in some women, early pregnancy. *See also* Morning sickness.

A simple case of "upset stomach" may disappear after one bout of vomiting. Longer or frequent vomiting bouts require medical attention.

Vulva. The outer lips of the vagina. *See also* Reproductive system, female.

Vulvar warts. Warts on the vulva may be caused by a virus spread from warts on fingers, or from a sexual partner's penis. The condition should be checked by a physician and treated with medication or removed.

Walleye. *See* Eye disorders, strabismus.

Wart, plantar. *See* Plantar wart.

Warts, genital. *See* Genital warts.

Wasting disease. A condition that affects people who have a serious progressive illness such as cancer or AIDS. Symptoms include fatigue, loss of appetite, weight loss, inability to concentrate, and apparent starvation.

Treatment consists of frequent small, nutritious, solid and liquid meals. In far advanced cases, or if a person cannot eat or drink normally, intravenous nourishment is provided.

Weight control. The maintenance of normal body weight, appropriate for one's height, weight, sex, and body frame. Normal body weight may go up or down by a few pounds over time. This is healthy and no cause for concern.

Problems may arise if a person loses or gains more than 10 to 15 percent of normal body weight, or switches between large weight gains and large weight losses.

Weight control is a major key to good health. If you stay in control of your weight you can avoid the health problems caused by over- or underweight. Prevent major weight changes with a healthy diet, regular exercise, and sufficient sleep. *See also* Body mass index; Food groups; Food pyramid.

Weight gain. An increase in body weight. While a small weight gain will not affect your health, problems may arise if you gain more than 10 to 15 percent of your normal body weight. Among other things, the extra weight places more stress on the knees. Fat is deposited in various body areas and may change a person's appearance.

A continuing gain in weight places strain on the heart. Excess fat intake may lead to the deposit of fatty plaques in blood vessels and may increase blood pressure. Over time, heart and blood vessel disease may develop. *See also* Body mass index; Food groups; Food pyramid; Weight control.

Weight loss. A decrease in body weight. If weight loss amounts to more than 10 to 15 percent of your total body weight, you need to see a doctor to find out why you are losing so much weight and how you can regain it.

Reasons for weight loss include illness with loss of appetite, strenuous exercise, fatigue, stress, poor dietary habits, and excessive dieting.

Girls who lose a lot of weight may have menstrual difficulties such as irregular periods, scant periods, or no periods. Great weight loss may be related to anorexia, a dangerous eating disorder. Medical attention and treatment are necessary to reverse this dangerous illness. *See also* Anorexia nervosa; Weight control.

Western blot test (WB). A blood test that confirms HIV infection by detecting HIV antibodies in the serum.

Wet dreams. *See* Nocturnal emission.

White blood cell, leukocyte (WBC). A component of blood. There are several different types of white blood cells—lymphocytes, monocytes, and others. Each type has a different function, from fighting infection to indicating the presence of an allergy.

Whiteheads. Inflamed skin areas with a white core, usually seen with acne. *See also* Acne; Pimples.

Whooping cough (pertussis). A dangerous, infectious respiratory disease that usually occurs during childhood. Adults can contract the disease if they did not have it as children, or were not vaccinated against it.

Cause: The organism *Borderella pertussis*.

Transmission: Inhalation of the infectious organisms sprayed in the air when the sick child coughs or sneezes.

Symptoms: Whooping cough begins with coldlike symptoms and a nighttime cough. After two weeks the ill person starts having severe coughing spells that end in a "whoop" sound, caused by breathing in quickly and deeply. Vomiting and choking may follow the coughing spells. The disease usually lasts about six weeks; in some cases it continues for two to three months.

Treatment: No specific treatment. The sick child or adult is made comfortable and given lots of fluids and frequent small meals.

Special precautions: Someone exposed to whooping cough may be able to avoid contracting the disease by taking antibiotics immediately after exposure and for about two weeks thereafter. Antibiotics will not help once symptoms are present. Immunizations given in infancy will prevent whooping cough and other infectious childhood diseases. Booster immunization shots, given at prescribed intervals, protect against these infections for life. *See also* Immunization.

Window period. The time during which a person may have contracted an infectious disease but as yet has no symptoms or positive test results.

Withdrawal method. A birth control technique in which the male removes his penis from his partner's vagina just before he ejaculates. The method is not as reliable as the Pill or condom. Even with very careful, prompt withdrawal, a few drops of semen may be expelled into the vagina and cause pregnancy.

Womb. Uterus. *See also* Reproductive system, female.

Wood's lamp. A special lamp used to determine the presence of a fungus infection on the scalp or skin. The lamp is also used to detect dried semen on the body of a person who has been raped or sexually assaulted in an attempted rape.

Works. Equipment such as syringes, needles, and pots (for boiling water), used by drug addicts to prepare drug solutions for injection into a vein.

X

X chromosome. Genetic material in sperm and egg cells that determines a baby's sex. Each egg and each sperm contains two sex chromosomes. Eggs carry two X chromosomes, which produce female sex characteristics. Sperm contain an X as well as a Y chromosome; the Y chromosome produces male sexual characteristics.

Once an egg is fertilized by a sperm, it begins to divide and multiply. Each of the new cells contains one sex chromosome from the sperm, and one from the egg. If both are X chromosomes, the baby will be a girl. If one is X and one is Y, the baby will be a boy. *See also* Chromosome; XX, XXY, XY, and Y chromosomes.

X rays (roentgen rays). Light rays that are passed through special equipment (an X-ray tube) that enables them to penetrate body tissues. Certain types of X rays are used to make a diagnosis; others are used to treat diseases such as cancer.

XX chromosomes. The usual gene combination in a female chromosome. *See also* Chromosome; Genes; X, XXY, XY, and Y chromosomes.

XXY chromosomes. An abnormal gene combination in male chromosomes. Boys born with this gene combination may develop Klinefelter's syndrome, a disease that causes sterility, enlarged breasts, and other physical abnormalities. *See also* Chromosome; Genes; X, XY, and Y chromosomes.

XY chromosome. The usual gene combination in a male. *See also* Chromosome; Genes; X, XX chromosomes.

Y

Y chromosome. A gene in male sperm. An egg fertilized with sperm that contains a Y chromosome will develop into a male baby. *See also* Chromosome; Genes; X, XX, XXY, and XY chromosomes.

Yeast infection. Infection caused by a fungus, a tiny plantlike organism. Common fungi include mildew and mushrooms. Some fungal types cause infections that can invade nearly every part of the body. The most commonly diagnosed yeast infection is the vaginal infection candidiasis, also known as moniliasis. *See also* Candidiasis.

Certain yeast infections occur only in people who have a defective immune system—for example, people who have AIDS.

Z

Zone, erogenous. *See* Erogenous zone.

Zoster, herpes. *See* Shingles.

Zygote. The fertilized egg before it begins to divide and multiply. *See also* Fertilization.

Appendixes

Appendix A
HOTLINES

Hotlines are useful resources when you need help in a hurry, if you want to talk about something confidential, or if you need a referral for a specific problem. Listed according to the problems they deal with, you will find the names, addresses, and telephone numbers of clinics, agencies, and organizations that can provide help and advice. You can dial 800 numbers free of charge, from anywhere in the United States.

Abortion and Family Planning
National Abortion Federation Hotline
1436 U Street NW
Washington, DC 20009
800-772-9100
9:30 A.M.–5:30 P.M. EST, Mon.–Fri.

Planned Parenthood
Planned Parenthood Clinics provide reproductive health services according to the individual's income. Teenagers can go to Planned Parenthood centers for birth control, pregnancy tests, STD testing and treatment, and abortion services and counseling. Look in your local telephone directory to find the nearest Planned Parenthood.

The Reproductive Health Technologies Project
800-584-9911
Information about emergency contraception and referrals to local services.

Abuse
Child abuse, domestic violence, sexual abuse

Childhelp USA
24-hour hotline: 800-4-A-CHILD
(For Spanish, press 2)

National Domestic Violence Hotline
24-hour hotline: 800-799-7233
(English/Spanish)
800-787-3224 (TDD)

AIDS
National Agencies
AIDS Hotline for Teens (TEENS.TAP)
800-234-8336
4 P.M.–8 P.M. EST, Mon.–Fri.

CDC National HIV and AIDS Hotline
800-342-AIDS (English)
800-344-SIDA (Spanish)
8 A.M.–2 A.M. EST, 7 days a week
800-243-7889 (TTY); 10 A.M.–10 P.M. EST, Mon.–Fri.

Teen AIDS Hotline
800-440-8336
6:00 P.M.–Midnight EST, Fri.–Sat.

Regional Agencies
CAYACC (Comprehensive Adolescent and Young Adult Care Center)
St. Luke's Roosevelt Hospital Center
1111 Amsterdam Avenue
New York, NY 10025
212-523-6301

Adolescent AIDS Program
Montefiore Medical Center
111 E. 210th Street
Bronx, NY 10467
718-882-0023
9 A.M.–5P.M., Mon.–Fri.; consultants on call

AIDS Action Committee
131 Clarendon Street
Boston, MA 02116

Information: 617-437-6200
Hotline: 617-450-1200
9 A.M.–9 P.M. EST, Mon.–Fri.

AID Atlanta
1430 W. Peachtree NW, Suite 100
Atlanta, GA 30309
InfoLine: 404-876-9944
Hotline: 404-872-0600
8:30 A.M.–5 P.M. EST, Mon.–Fri.

AIDS Project Los Angeles
1313 North Vine
Los Angeles, CA 90046
213-876-AIDS/800-822-2437 (CA only)
9 A.M.–9 P.M., 7 days a week

Aliveness Project Center for Living
730 E. 38th Street
Minneapolis, MN 55407
Information: 621-822-7946
24-hour hotline: 612-822-0826

Neon Street Programs
4822 North Broadway, 2nd Floor
Chicago, IL 60640
312-271-6366
8:30 A.M.–8:30 P.M., 7 days a week

Pediatric and Pregnancy AIDS Hotline
Albert Einstein College of Medicine
1300 Morris Park Avenue
Bronx, NY 10467
718-430-3333

Alcohol Abuse
AL-ANON and ALA-TEEN Family
Headquarters
800-356-9996
9 A.M.–5:30 P.M., Mon.–Fri.
Provides counseling and services for family
members of alcoholics, teenagers of alcoholic
parents, and teenage alcoholics. Check telephone directory for the local chapter.

Focus on Recovery:
Alcohol/Drug Abuse Hotline
24-hour hotline: 800-222-0828

Youth Crisis Hotline for Teens
800-448-4663

Alcoholics Anonymous
307 Seventh Avenue
New York, NY 10001
212-647-1680
9 A.M.–10 P.M., Mon.–Fri.

ASAP Family Treatment Center
P.O. Box 6150
Malibu, CA 90264-6150
24-hour hotline: 800-367-2727

Families Anonymous, Inc.
P.O. Box 548
Van Nuys, CA 91408
For families of alcoholics; will refer you to a
local family service office

National Association for Children of
Alcoholics
Suite 100
11426 Rockville Pike
Rockville, MD 20852
301-468-0985

National Council on Alcoholism and
Drug Dependence Hope Line
24-hour hotline: 800-622-2255 (touch-tone
phone only)

Allergies
National Institute of Allergy and Infectious
Diseases
Office of Communications
Health Bldg. 31, Rm. 7A-32
Bethesda, MD 20892
301-496-5717
8:30 A.M.–5 P.M., Mon.–Fri.

Arthritis
Arthritis Foundation
800-283-7800

National Arthritis and Musculoskeletal and
Skin Diseases Information Clearinghouse
9000 Rockville Pike

A

Building 31, Room 9AO4
Bethesda, MD 20892
301-495-4484
Supports multipurpose arthritis centers around the country. Provides publications and information about community services.

Asthma

Allergy and Asthma Network/Mothers of Asthmatics, Inc.
800-878-4403

American Lung Association
800-LUNG-USA
Will reach lung association in your state.

Asthma and Allergy Foundation of America
800-7-ASTHMA

Cancer

All agencies and organizations can refer you to local support groups.

American Cancer Society
800-ACS-2345

Cancer Care Inc.
Social Services Department
1180 Avenue of Americas
New York, NY 10036
212-221-3300
9 A.M.–5 P.M., Mon.–Fri.

Cancer Information Service
800-4-CANCER (English/Spanish)
Answers cancer-related questions. Center is also a good source for pamphlets and other information.

Leukemia Society of America, Inc.
600 Third Avenue
New York, NY 10016
24-hour hotline: 800-955-4LSA

Share (Self-Help for Women with Breast and Ovarian Cancer)
1501 Broadway, Suite 1720
New York, NY 10036
Information: 212-260-0580

24-hour hotlines: 212-382-2111 (English); 212-719-4454 (Spanish)
Refers to local support groups.

Candlelighters Childhood Cancer Foundation
7910 Woodmont Avenue, Suite 460
Bethesda, MD 20814-3015
Information, service, and support groups for children and adolescents with cancer and their families

Depression

Family Services of America
Agencies in every major city in the United States and offers low-cost family counseling and special teen rap groups. Check telephone directory for the local Family Service office.

National Depressive and Manic-Depressive Association (NDMDA)
730 North Franklin, Suite 501
Chicago, IL 60610
800-82NDMDA
Provides information about teenage depression and provides referrals for local physicians who can help.

Diabetes

American Diabetes Association
P.O. Box 25757
1660 Duke St.
Alexandria, VA 22314
800–342–2383

Juvenile Diabetes Foundation International
432 Park Avenue South
New York, NY 10016
800-223-1138

Digestive Disorders

American Liver and Hepatitis Foundation
1425 Pompton Avenue
Cedar Grove, NJ 07009
24-hour hotline: 800-223-0179

Crohn's and Colitis Foundation of America
444 Park Avenue South, 11th Floor
New York, NY 10016
800-343-3537

National Digestive Diseases Information
Clearinghouse
2 Information Way
Bethesda, MD 20892-3570
301-654-3810

Disabilities
National Information Center for Youth with
Disabilities
800–695-0295 (also TDD access)
9:30 A.M.–5:30 P.M. EST, Mon.–Fri.

Drug Abuse
(See listings under Alcohol Abuse)

Dyslexia and Learning Disabilities
Learning Disabilities Hotline
212-605-6730

Learning Disabilities Association of
America
4156 Library Road
Pittsburg, PA 15234
412-341-1515

Eating Disorders
American Anorexia and Bulimia Association
293 Central Park West, Suite 1R
New York, NY 10024
212-501-8351
9 A.M.–5 P.M., Mon.–Fri.

Anorexia Nervosa and Related Eating
Disorders
P.O. Box 102
Eugene, OR 97405
503-344-1144

National Eating Disorders Organization
6655 South Yale
Tulsa, OK 74136
918-481-4044
8 A.M.–12 P.M. CST, Mon.–Fri.

National Association of Anorexia Nervosa
and Associated Disorders (ANAD)
P.O. Box 7
Highland Park, IL 60035
847-831-3438
9 A.M.–5 P.M. CST, Mon.–Fri.

Epilepsy
Epilepsy Foundation of America
4351 Garden City Drive
Landover, MD 20785-2267
800-332-1000

Family Planning
Planned Parenthood (see under Abortion and
Family Planning)

Gay and Lesbian Services
Gay Switchboard Hotline
215-546-7100 (Philadelphia only)
7 P.M.–10 P.M., Sun.–Tues.
6 P.M.–11 P.M., Wed.–Sat.

Gay and Lesbian Anti-Violence Project
212-807-0197 (New York City only)

National Gay Task Force
Crisis Line 800-227-7044

Parents, Families, and Friends of Lesbians
and Gays, Inc.
1012 14th Street, NW, Suite 700
Washington, D.C. 20005
202-638-4200

Sexuality Information and Education
Council of the United States (SIECUS)
30 West 42nd Street, Suite 350
New York, NY 10036
212-819-9770
9 A.M.–5 P.M., Mon.–Fri.

Hearing Impaired Services
Crisis Hotline for the Hearing Impaired
Deaf Emergency TDD
If you are in an emergency situation and
need an emergency operator, there is a local

A

listing on the cover of your telephone directory.

Lupus Erythematosus
Lupus Foundation of America
4 Research Place
Rockville, MD 20850
800-74-LUPUS

Multiple Sclerosis
Multiple Sclerosis Association of America
760 Haddenfield Road
Cherry Hill, NJ 08002
800-LEARNMS

Poison Control Center
See listing of area number on the inside cover of the Telephone Directory.

Psoriasis
National Psoriasis Foundation
P.O. Box 9009
Portland, OR 97223-7195
24-hour hotline: 800-723-9166

Rape
Rape Crisis Center
800-352-7273

Sex Crime Report Line
Call your local police department. It will transfer your call.

Runaway and Homeless Teenagers
National Runaway Hotline
24-hour hotline: 800-621-4000
Counseling and referrals for runaways and homeless teens

Sexuality
Sexuality Information and Education Council of the United States (SIECUS)
30 West 42nd Street, Suite 350
New York, NY 10036
212-819-9770
9 A.M.–5 P.M., Mon.–Fri.

Sexually Transmitted Diseases (STDs)
CDC National Sexually Transmitted Diseases Hotline
800-227-8922
8 A.M.–11 P.M. EST, Mon.–Fri.

Planned Parenthood (see Abortion and Family Planning) provides information and STD treatment.

Sickle Cell Disease
National Sickle Cell Disease Program
National Heart, Lung, and Blood Institute
Room 508, Federal Building
7550 Wisconsin Avenue
Bethesda, MD 20892
301-496-6931

Sickle Cell Disease Association of America
200 Corporate Point, Suite 495
Culver City, CA 90230-7633
800-421-8453

Suicide
American Association of Suicidology
2459 South Ash
Denver, CO 80222
303-692-0985

National Commision on Youth Suicide Prevention
67 Irving Place South
New York, NY 10003
212-532-2400

Samaritans: Suicide Services
500 Commonwealth Avenue
Boston, MA 02215
24-hour hotline: 617-247-0220

Tuberculosis
American Lung Association
800-LUNG-USA
Will reach lung association in your state.

Appendix B

MEDICATIONS AND THEIR USE IN TEEN HEALTH CARE

Modern medicines, taken correctly, can cure illnesses, relieve pain, hasten recovery, and improve the quality of life. They come in many forms: as liquids to be swallowed, or to be instilled by the drop in eyes and ears; as solids, in pills or tablets taken by mouth; as medicated creams, ointments, or patches applied to the skin; or as suppositories inserted into the rectum or vagina. Some medications are inhaled through the nose to relieve breathing and other problems. Certain drugs cannot be taken by mouth because stomach juices inactivate them or because the drug's effects are needed quickly to save a patient's life. These drugs are injected into a muscle or vein to get them into the bloodstream almost immediately.

Two types of drugs are available legally: over-the-counter drugs (OTCs), which you can buy in any drugstore; and prescription drugs (available only with a doctor's prescription), which are generally stronger and often more dangerous than OTC drugs. Doctors are familiar with the chemical composition, benefits, and adverse effects of each drug they prescribe. The doctor prescribes it only after:

1. Examining the patient and making a diagnosis;
2. Determining the drug needed to treat the patient's condition;
3. Calculating the correct dosage and deciding for how long the drug should be used;

4. Checking the patient for allergies that might cause a dangerous reaction. If a patient is sensitive to one drug, another medication is prescribed.

In this Appendix, drugs are grouped by treatment purpose, with examples of OTC and prescription drugs available in each category. The list includes many commonly used and prescribed drugs. It is not a comprehensive listing of all available drugs, and there is no intention to recommend any particular drug.

If you develop any symptoms of illness, don't treat yourself. A doctor or health care clinic should determine the treatment you need.

Acne Medications

Purpose: To open up skin pores or clear up infections.

OTC drugs: Oxy-5, Oxy-10.

Prescription drugs: Lotions, creams, or gels. Benzoyl peroxide, Retin-A, Accutane (pills). (Important caution: do not take Accutane if any possibility of pregnancy exists.)

Prescription antibiotic drugs that reduce bacteria that cause inflammation: Pills—Erythromycin, Minocin. Topical solutions—Cleocin-T, T-stat, Erycette.

Analgesics, Pain Relievers

Purpose: To lessen or eliminate pain. Except for chronic problems, pain is usually temporary. If pain persists, a doctor should be consulted. Stopping pain medication as soon as acute pain disappears prevents dependence on unneeded medicines.

OTC drugs: Aspirin, Tylenol (acetaminophen), Advil (ibuprofen).

Prescription drugs: Anaprox, Naprosyn, Motrin.

For severe pain, such as after surgery or an injury, a doctor may prescribe a narcotic drug. These drugs are prescribed with special care because their use may be habit forming.

Codeine, a relatively mild narcotic drug, is often combined with Tylenol for relief of moderate pain. Stronger narcotics include Demerol and morphine. Narcotic drugs are generally prescribed in an emergency room, clinic, or hospital so their use can be supervised for adverse effects. They are discontinued as soon as possible so patients will not become dependent on their use.

Antacid Drugs

Purpose: To counteract excess stomach acid.

OTC drugs: Mylanta, Maalox, Alka-Seltzer, Tagamet HB, Pepcid AC.

Prescription drugs: Prilosec, Tagamet, Pepcid.

Antianxiety Drugs

Purpose: To lessen or relieve anxiety or nervousness.

OTC drugs: None.

Prescription drugs: Atarax, Librium, Valium, Xanax.

Antibiotic Drugs

Purpose: To treat infections by killing or inhibiting the growth of harmful bacteria and other organisms.

OTC drugs: Neosporin and bacitracin ointments (to treat skin infections).

Prescription drugs: Penicillin group—ampicillin, amoxicillin, dicloxacillin.

Cephalosporin group—Keflex, Velosef, Ceclor.

Macrolide group (used for people allergic to penicillin)—erythromycin, Eryc, Biaxin, Zithromax.

Tetracycline group—tetracycline, doxycycline, Minocin.

Quinolone group—ciprofloxacin, norfloxacin, Maxaquin.

Nitrofurantoin group—Macrodantin.

Sulfa drug group—Gantrisin, Bactrim DS, Septra DS.

Zithromax—a one-time treatment for chlamydial infection. Also used for bronchitis (longer treatment period).

Anticonstipation Drugs *See* Laxatives.

Antidepressant Drugs

Purpose: To treat depression.

OTC drugs: None.

Prescription drugs: Elavil, Pamelor, Paxil, Prozac, Tofranil, Wellbutrin, Zoloft.

Antidiarrheal Drugs

Purpose: To stop diarrhea.

OTC drugs: Pepto-Bismol, Imodium.

Prescription drugs: Lomotil.

Antifungal Drugs

Purpose: To kill or inhibit the growth of fungi or yeast organisms.

OTC drugs: Lotrimin for skin infections, Tinactin for athlete's foot, Gyne-lotrimin and Monistat for vaginal infections.

Prescription drugs: Nizoral and Spectazole for skin infections, Nizoral and Spectazole for athlete's foot, Terazol for vaginal infections, Diflucan for vaginal infections or thrush.

Antihistamine (Allergy) Drugs

Purpose: To counter symptoms of an allergic reaction, such as congestion, swelling, itching, and hives.

OTC drugs: Benadryl, Chlor-Trimeton.

Prescription drugs: Atarax, Seldane, Hismanal, Claritin, epinephrine in a bee sting kit (a prefilled syringe and needle for immediate self-injection).

Antinausea Drugs

Purpose: To stop nausea or vomiting.

OTC drugs: Benadryl, Dramamine.

Prescription drugs: Atarax, Compazine, Tigan.

Antipruritic (Anti-itch) Drugs

Purpose: To relieve itching caused by a rash, allergy, or skin disease.

OTC drugs: Calamine, Cortaid, Lanacane.

Prescription drugs: hydrocortisone 1%, hydrocortisone 2.5%, Valisone 0.1%, Lidex, Kenalog.

Antipsychotic Drugs

Purpose: To treat severe mental disorders.

OTC drugs: None.

Prescription drugs: Clozaril, Haldol, Mellaril, Stelazine, Thorazine.

Antituberculosis Drugs

Purpose: To cure tuberculosis.

OTC drugs: None.

Prescription drugs: Isoniazid, rifampin, ethambutol, streptomycin.

Antiviral Drugs

Purpose: To treat viral infections.

OTC drugs: None.

Prescription drugs: Amantadine, Zovirax.

Asthma Medications

Purpose: To relieve wheezing and shortness of breath.

OTC drugs: Primatene mist, tablets (for use only if no doctor available; get medical treatment as soon as possible).

Prescription drugs: Inhalers to relax tight breathing tubes—Proventil, Alupent, Ventolin.

Inhalers to prevent or decrease swelling of the breathing tubes—Intal, Azmacort.

Long-lasting inhalant drug that dilates breathing tubes (bronchodilator). Used twice daily. Caution: Do not use for an asthmatic emergency as the drug does not take effect for 30 to 60 minutes after use—Serevent.

Pills to relax tight breathing tubes—Proventil, Alupent, Ventolin.

Pills to prevent or decrease swelling of the breathing tubes—prednisone.

Cold and Cough Remedies (Decongestants)

Purpose: To clear up a stuffy nose (nasal congestion) and relieve cough.

OTC drugs: For colds—nasal sprays such as Afrin, pills such as Sudafed, Actifed.

For coughs—Robitussin, Benylin, Tuss-Ornade.

Prescription drugs: For colds—Entex LA, Trinalin, Deconsal II.

For coughs—Hycodan, phenergan with codeine, Tessalon Perles.

Contraceptive Medications

Purpose: To prevent pregnancy.

OTC drugs: None.

Oral contraceptives: Birth control pills (the Pill). Birth control pills come in several types: Monophasic, biphasic, and triphasic. Each type contains a somewhat different combination of female hormones. The Pill must be taken every day during the menstrual cycle in order to prevent pregnancy. Frequently used oral contraceptive pills include Brevicon, Demulen, Levlen, Loestrin, Lo/Ovral, Norinyl, Ortho-Novum, Tri-Norinyl, and Triphasil.

Injectable contraceptive medications: Depo-Provera contraceptive injection. Effective for three months. Must then be repeated for continued protection against pregnancy.

Implant contraceptive medications: The Norplant System. Six flexible closed

B

capsules are implanted (surgically inserted) under the skin of the upper arm. The capsules contain the female progestin. Norplant is effective for up to five years. It can then be removed and replaced by new capsules.

Diabetic Medications

Purpose: To provide the body with insulin, a hormone necessary for proper digestion and sugar metabolism.

OTC drugs: None.

Prescription drugs: Pills—Diabinese, Glucotrol, Micronase.

Insulin (must be injected)—regular insulin, NPH insulin, Lente insulin, Ultra-lente insulin, Humulin.

Fade Creams

Purpose: To lighten pigmented blotches on the skin.

OTC fade drugs: Esoterica.

Prescription drugs: Solaquine Forte, Eldopaque Forte.

Iron Drugs

Purpose: To treat iron deficiency, anemia.

OTC drugs: Slow Fe, ferrous sulfate, ferrous gluconate.

Prescription drugs: Feosol.

Laxatives

Purpose: To relieve constipation (insufficient or hard bowel movements).

OTC drugs: Fiberall, Metamucil, Ex-Lax.

Prescription drugs: Senokot.

Seizure (Antiepilepsy) Drugs

Purpose: To stop or prevent seizures.

OTC drugs: None.

Prescription drugs: Depakene, Dilantin, phenobarbital, Tegretol.

Skin Moisturizers (Emollients)

Purpose: To decrease skin dryness.

OTC products: Vaseline Intensive Care, Nivea, Alpha Keri lotions, and a wide range of products of cosmetic companies.

Prescription preparations: Lac-Hydrin lotion.

Steroid Drugs

Purpose: To reduce inflammation (irritation, swelling) on the surface of and inside the body.

OTC drugs: Cream or lotion—Calecort and Cortaid.

Prescription drugs: Cream or lotion—hydrocortisone 1%, hydrocortisone 2.5%, Valisone 0.1%, Lidex, Kenalog.

Pills—Prednisone, Decadron.

Vitamins

Purpose: To provide ingredients essential for maintaining health and aiding the body's metabolism.

OTC preparations: Multivitamins—One-a-day, Centrum.

Prescription preparations: Berocca Plus.

Appendix C

STREET DRUGS—WHAT YOU NEED TO KNOW ABOUT THEM

Drugs you buy over the counter or by prescription are usually intended to cure, or at least relieve, pain, an infection, or other illness, or to help maintain or restore health. Drug companies carefully monitor their production to make sure the ingredients are pure, have the required strength, and are not contaminated.

Other drugs, some of them illegal, serve no useful purpose and may do serious damage to the body. People who use these drugs expect them to:

- Solve their problems of growing up—for example, to have more friends, to cope with anger or frustration, or to have better relationships;
- Make them forget their problems;
- Take away painful feelings—for example, after the breakup of a friendship;
- Give them a high—a feeling that they are on top of the world;
- Help them to have better or more frequent sex.

Many of these substances cause permanent damage to vital organs. Some can cause death very quickly. They contain chemicals that may stimulate or depress vital body systems, such as the heart and lungs, to a point where the body can't cope. The results may be fatal.

Legally available substances such as alcohol and cigarettes also undermine a user's health. Alcohol damages the liver and other major organs and impairs judgment. Heavy drinking over time may cause cancer. Cigarettes are harmful to the heart, the blood vessels, and the respiratory system. Long-term smoking often causes lung cancer. Moreover, cigarettes also harm nonsmokers who inhale the smoke, including family members, friends, and coworkers. Studies also show that children of smokers develop asthma more readily and have more asthma attacks.

Illegal drugs and substances (street drugs), such as marijuana, cocaine, crack, and heroin, are manufactured without controls or supervision by a qualified agency. They may be stronger or weaker than expected, and they may be contaminated by dirty or toxic substances.

Some people think they are safe and in control if they merely smoke a joint or take an upper now and then. But the high and the other effects of a drug last only for a while. After that, the user may feel worse. Users may find themselves wanting larger amounts of drugs and under pressure to get money to support their growing habit. Some will commit crimes to get money. Buying, possessing, using, or selling illegal drugs are also crimes, and can result in fines or imprisonment.

The list below includes the most often abused drugs—both legal and illegal—along with each drug's effects. Street names, real names, and terms used in connection with drug and substance abuse are also included.

C

The names of street drugs change frequently, and vary by area.

SEDATIVES (HYPNOTICS)

Sedatives, in small quantities, make you feel relaxed and easy. Moderate amounts make you feel sleepy. Large amounts may result in coma (deep unconsciousness) or death.

Alcohol. Wine, wine coolers, beer, malt liquor, rum, whiskey, vodka, gin, and others
Appearance: Clear or colored liquid taken by mouth
Desired effects: Release of inhibitions, mild euphoria, happy feelings
Harmful effects: Nausea, vomiting, poor coordination, slurred speech, drowsiness, coma, death; liver damage after long-term use
Beer is probably the most common alcoholic drug of abuse, particularly among high school and college students.

About 82 percent of high school students report using alcohol on occasion. At first, alcohol may be used only occasionally. Larger amounts and more frequent drinking follow. Binge-drinkers down a number of drinks quickly. Binge-drinking is especially dangerous if strong alcoholic beverages are used.

A teen who binge-drinks rapidly becomes intoxicated. With continued drinking, the teen may pass out and die. Young people who drive after binge-drinking may be involved in accidents. A California study revealed that in more than one-third of all fatal car accidents involving teenagers, the driver had taken one or more drugs—most often alcohol.

Barbiturates. Goofballs, downers, blues, yellow jackets, red birds, red devils, rainbows
Appearance: Blue, yellow, red, or multicolored pills, taken by mouth
Desired effects: Release of inhibitions, mild euphoria, relaxation
Harmful side effects: Drowsiness, slow breathing, mental confusion, slurred speech, coma, death

Some people start with a prescription for barbiturate to help them sleep. After a while, they may need more and more of the drug. In time they are hooked (dependent); they can't fall asleep without the drug.

People who use stimulants such as cocaine or amphetamines may also use barbiturates to cut down unpleasant side effects, such as nervousness or shakiness.

Methaqualone (Quaaludes). Ludes, love drug, wallbangers
Appearance: White crystals that can be dissolved in alcohol or water
Method of use: Usually taken by mouth in a tablet or capsule but sometimes smoked
Desired effects: A pleasant high, reduced inhibitions, increased self-confidence, sleepiness
Harmful effects: numbness and tingling, slurred speech, muscle spasms, feelings of losing one's mind, increased heart rate, chills or sweating, slow breathing, and with overdose, coma or death

HALLUCINOGENS

Hallucinogens alter a person's perception of reality. The user may believe it's possible to leap out of a window and not get hurt. Hallucinogens may also change a person's mood and affect the ability to think clearly and make sensible decisions.

Ketimine. Special-K
Appearance: A white powder
Desired effects: Euphoria, hallucinations
Harmful effects: Similar to LSD. Hallucinations may be terrifying; increased heart rate and blood pressure; may lead to circulatory collapse, shock, and death.
Note: Ketimine is used as an anesthetic drug in a hospital setting, under medical supervision.

LSD (Lysergic acid diethylamide). Acid, snoopy, cube, lid, blotter, windowpane
Appearance: A white powder usually dis-

solved in water and sprinkled on sugar cubes, blotting paper, or tablets

Method of use: Taken by mouth, inhaled, or injected

Desired effects: Senses may become temporarily sharper—colors seem brighter, odors more pungent, sounds louder.

Users may feel lighter than air, or as if they are having a religious experience.

Harmful effects: Anxiety, depression, mental confusion, terrifying hallucinations, increased body temperature, chills, shivering, rapid breathing

Later harmful effects: Flashbacks of experiences from an earlier episode of drug use

Marijuana. Weed, joint, grass, ganja, reefer

Appearance: Powder or dried leaves

Method of use: Smoking

Desired effects: Feelings of well-being, a high, drowsiness, relaxation, enhanced senses (more acute hearing, vision, taste)

Harmful effects: Cough, bronchitis, asthma, memory loss, loss of interest, decreased concentration, impaired coordination

Mescaline. Mesc

Appearance: A white powder, usually sold in capsules

Method of use: Usually taken by mouth, sometimes sprinkled on tobacco or marijuana and smoked, occasionally dissolved and injected

Desired effects: Same effects as LSD

Harmful effects: Same as LSD

PCP (Phencyclidine). Angel dust

Appearance: A white powder usually dissolved in water or alcohol, packed in pills, or placed in capsules

Method of use: Taken orally, snorted, smoked if sprinkled on a marijuana cigarette, sometimes injected

Desired effects: Relaxation, feeling of floating, slowing down of time, feeling high

Harmful effects: Blurred vision, dizziness, drowsiness, increased blood pressure and breathing rate, confusion, restlessness, panic, terror, violent behavior, convulsions, coma, death

NARCOTICS

This class of drugs is very effective in reducing or relieving physical and emotional pain. Narcotics can also produce euphoria. In larger doses they cause drowsiness.

Heroin. Horse, white lady, smack, China white

Appearance: White powder

Method of use: Usually dissolved in boiling water and injected under the skin (skin popping) or injected into a vein (mainlining), sometimes snorted or smoked.

Desired effects: Relief of pain, euphoria

Harmful side effects: Nausea, vomiting, decreased physical activity, inability to concentrate, lowered blood pressure, shallow breathing, coma, death

Methadone. Meth

Appearance: White crystalline powder dissolved in water or alcohol

Method of use: By mouth or by injection

Desired effects: Pain relief, euphoria, relaxation, drowsiness

Harmful effects: Deep sleep, coma

Methadone is frequently used in drug treatment programs. It relieves the addict's intense craving for drugs such as heroin. Methadone produces a feeling of well-being, but less euphoria in addicts than in nonaddicts. Under medical supervision, the drug allows addicts to feel well enough so they can live without heroin.

Morphine. Morph

Appearance: A white powder that can be dissolved in water or alcohol

Method of use: By mouth in the form of pills or by injection

Desired effects: Relief of pain, drowsiness, relaxation, euphoria

Harmful effects: Lowered blood pressure, slow breathing and heart rate, coma, death

Morphine is very effective in relieving pain, particularly after surgery or after an accident. Its use is carefully monitored and controlled and this type of short-term use rarely results in dependence or addiction.

When used as a street drug, there is no monitoring or control of effects. It is used to get high and is taken in much larger doses than are prescribed for pain relief. The result may be coma and death.

Street morphine's effectiveness can be higher or lower than expected, as its production was not monitored. The street drug may also be contaminated, causing infection at the injection site.

STIMULANTS

Stimulants produce a feeling of great well-being (euphoria). Small amounts may reduce hunger pangs and enhance alertness. Larger amounts may cause the heart to beat rapidly and blood pressure to rise to very high levels.

Amphetamines. Uppers, bennies, black beauties, crystal, speed, hearts, Christmas trees

Appearance: Usually in pill form; also sold as a white powder to be mixed with water or alcohol

Method of use: By mouth in liquid or pill form; may also be injected

Desired effects: Euphoria, reduced appetite, increased energy

Harmful effects: Headache, increased heart rate, increased blood pressure, chest pain, fainting, seizures, coma, death

Caffeine

Appearance: A white powder; occurs naturally in chocolate, tea, coffee, some soft drinks, and sometimes is added to substances

Method of use: Taken by mouth

Desired effects: Increased alertness, reduced fatigue

Harmful effects: Insomnia, increased heart rate and blood pressure

Cocaine. Coke, flake, snow, rock, crack

Appearance: White powder or small white pellets

Method of use: May be snorted, rubbed onto gums, smoked, injected

Desired effects: Sense of well-being, euphoria, reduced appetite, increased energy, enhanced feeling of power

Harmful effects: Depression once the euphoria has worn off; anxiety, headache, paranoia, increased heart rate and blood pressure, fainting, heart attack, seizures, coma, death after continued use or use of large quantities

Crack. *See* Cocaine.

Nicotine

Appearance: An oily liquid extracted from the leaf of the tobacco plant and processed into a white or colorless crystal

Method of use: Chewed, snorted, smoked

Desired effects: Increased alertness, relaxation, temporary suppression of appetite

Harmful effects: Cough, upper respiratory tract infections, bronchitis, cancer of the tongue, throat and lungs, narrowing of blood vessels leading to heart damage.

STREET DRUGS AND DRUG TERMS

Acapulco Gold. A type of marijuana grown in Mexico.

Acid. LSD (lysergic acid diethylamide), lids, snoopies, blotter, windowpane.

Alkies. Alcoholics.

Angel Dust. PCP (phencyclidine).

Baby-sit. Guide someone through a first drug experience.

Back to back. Smoking crack after injecting heroin, or using heroin after smoking crack.

Backtrack. Allow blood to flow back into a needle during injection.

Bad trip. An unpleasant drug experience, usually after using LSD.

Bag. How a street drug, usually marijuana, is packaged. A trey bag is an amount of marijuana sold for three dollars; a nickel bag is sold for five dollars.

Bazooka. Cocaine, crack.

Beaming. Feeling high.

Beam me up, Scottie. Crack dipped in PCP.

Bennies. Amphetamines or speed.

Big 40. A 40-ounce bottle of beer.

Binge. Using excessive amounts of drugs for a period of time.

Black beauties. Amphetamines.

Blow. Cocaine.

Blunt. A large marijuana cigarette or a hollowed-out cigar filled with marijuana.

Bogart a joint. Salivate on a marijuana cigarette or refuse to share.

Brick. A compressed block of opium, morphine, or hashish.

Buddha. Marijuana.

Bummer. A bad experience with drugs; a bad trip.

Buzz. Feeling high, usually after alcohol or marijuana use.

Chicken scratching. Searching on hands and knees for crack.

China white. A type of heroin from Asia.

Cisco. Alcohol (a brand of wine); cheap wine with high alcohol content.

Coke. Cocaine.

Cold turkey. Sudden withdrawal from drugs without medications.

Colt 45. Alcohol, a brand of malt liquor.

Come down. The flip side of beaming; the physical and psychological letdown after a drug has worn off.

Connection. A supplier of drugs.

Contact. A secondhand way of getting high, as when a nonsmoker experiences some of the drug's effects by inhaling other people's marijuana-laced smoke.

Cop. To obtain drugs.

Crack. A crystallized form of cocaine that can be smoked; leads to a quick, intense high of short duration, followed by a period of depression.

Crash. The come-down or period of depression experienced after taking a drug.

Crazy Horse. Alcohol (brand of beer).

Crystal. A type of methamphetamine, a stimulant drug.

Cube. A sugar cube laced with LSD.

Cut. To dilute a drug, usually heroin.

Deal. A sale of drugs.

Dealer. A person who sells street drugs.

Dope. Drugs in general; also an expression of excellence, "That was real dope!"

Downers. Barbiturates.

Drop. To take a lid of acid.

Dust. Angel dust (PCP).

E. Ecstasy pills.

Ecstasy. MDMA, a drug related to amphetamines; a drug used for its sexually stimulating (aphrodisiac) effects.

Fiend. A drug abuser.

Fix. Taking drugs to fill a physical or psychological craving.

Flip out. To have a psychological reaction to a drug—for example, hallucinate or "go crazy."

Freak. A person who will do anything to obtain drugs; similar to a fiend.

Getting burned. Buying drugs of poor quality, such as heroin that has been diluted or cut.

Goofball. Barbiturate.

Gorilla biscuits. PCP.

Grass. Marijuana.

Half-moon. Half pill.

Hash. Hashish, a narcotic drug.

Head. The extent of a person's high, as in "How's your head?"; or a heavy drug user, as an "acid head."

Herb. Marijuana.

High. Temporary feeling of happiness (euphoria) after taking certain drugs.

Hit. Taking a certain amount of a drug.

C

Hype. A hypodermic needle; or an expression of excellence, as in "that was real hype."

Joint, J. A marijuana cigarette.

Kilo. A metric measurement equal to 2.2 pounds of a drug.

King Cobra. Alcohol, brand of beer.

Lace. To add another compound or chemical to a drug. Heroin, for example, can be laced with strychnine, a poison that causes serious complications.

Laughing gas. Nitrous oxide, which causes a feeling of euphoria when inhaled.

Line. A quantity of cocaine.

Love drug. Methaqualone.

LSD. Lysergic acid diethylamide.

Ludes. Quaaludes, a sedative drug similar to barbiturates.

Mesc. Mescaline, a hallucinogenic drug similar in action to LSD.

Moon. Pill.

Munchies. A craving for food while smoking marijuana.

Mushroom ('Shrooms). A type of fungus that, when ingested, can sometimes create a hallucinogenic effect similar to that of LSD.

OD. An overdose, a physical complication after taking too much of a drug; may result in death.

On the nod. Under the influence of narcotics or depressants.

Opium. A narcotic drug.

PCP. Phencyclidine.

Poppers. Amyl nitrite.

Pot. Marijuana.

Rainbows (Tuinal, tueys). A type of barbiturate.

Reds. Amphetamines.

Reefers. Marijuana cigarettes.

Ripped. High.

Ripped off. Stuck with bad drugs; or robbed of drugs.

Roach. The small remnant of a marijuana cigarette.

Roach clip. A device used to hold a remnant of marijuana cigarette.

Rock star. Female who trades sex for crack or for money to buy crack.

Roll. The process of making a marijuana cigarette.

Run. Similar to a binge.

Rush. A rapid high.

Scratch. Money.

Skeezer. A prostitute on crack.

Snoopy. Acid placed on a cartoon figure decal.

Snow. Cocaine.

Spaced. High.

Speed. Amphetamine.

Speedball. Heroin and cocaine.

Speed freak. Amphetamine addict.

Stash. A supply of drugs.

Step on. To dilute or cut a drug.

St. Ides. Alcohol, a brand of beer.

Stoned. High; out of it.

Straight. Not using drugs; clean.

Strung out. Addicted to drugs.

Tab. A small quantity of acid.

THC. Tetrahydrocannabinol, the active ingredient in marijuana and hashish.

Toasted. Get high.

Toke. To inhale while smoking a marijuana cigarette.

Totaled. High, wiped out, unable to function.

Trip. The experience of getting high; also called a ride.

Uppers. Amphetamines.

Wallbanger. Methaqualone.

Wasted. High, unable to function.

White girl. Cocaine; heroin.

Wired. Intense anxiety after using amphetamines or cocaine.

Works. Equipment used to inject drugs: a syringe, needle, a tourniquet, matches, and a spoon.

Wrecked. High.

X. Ecstasy pills.

Zonked. High.

Appendix D
HEALTH CARE SPECIALISTS

Adolescent medicine specialist (Ephebiatrician). A physician who treats problems of teenagers.

Allergist. A physician who treats people who have allergies.

Anesthesiologist. A physician who gives anesthesia to people undergoing surgery and who may also treat severe pain problems.

Audiologist. A health professional who tests and evaluates hearing.

Cardiologist. A physician who treats diseases of the heart.

Cardiothoracic surgeon. A physician who performs surgery for heart and blood vessel diseases.

Chiropractor. A medical specialist who uses manipulation of the spine to improve medical conditions, such as lower back pain.

Dentist. A health professional who treats problems of the teeth.

Dermatologist. A physician who treats skin diseases.

Dietitian (nutritionist). A specialist who prescribes appropriate diets for healthy children and adults, for people with conditions such as obesity or underweight, or diseases that require special diets as a part of treatment.

Ear, nose, and throat specialist (otorhinolaryngologist). A physician who treats ear, nose, and throat problems.

Endocrinologist. A physician who treats glandular disorders.

Endodontist. A dentist who specializes in treating root canal and related dental problems.

Family doctor. A physician who takes care of the medical problems of adults and children.

Ephebiatrician. *See* Adolescent medicine specialist.

Gastroenterologist. A physician who treats diseases of the digestive system.

General practitioner. A physician who treats a wide range of medical problems.

Geneticist. A physician or other scientist who researches and analyzes inherited conditions and diseases and who counsels prospective parents about the likelihood of transmitting them to their children.

Geriatrician. A physician who treats the medical problems of elderly people.

Gynecologist. A physician who cares for women's health and treats diseases of the female reproductive system.

Hematologist. A physician who treats diseases of the blood and the blood-forming organs.

Home health aide. A person trained to give physical care at home to people who are unable to care for themselves.

Internist. A physician who specializes in treating medical diseases of adults.

Licensed practical nurse (LPN). *See* Nurse.

Medical office assistant. A health care worker who performs clerical and laboratory tasks in a physician's office.

Neonatologist. A physician who takes care of premature infants and newborn infants with medical problems.

Nephrologist. A physician who treats diseases of the kidneys and urinary tract.

Neurologist. A physician who treats problems of the nervous system.

Neurosurgeon. A physician who specializes in treating people with problems of the nervous system that require surgery.

Nurse. A person who has been educated to provide health care and to dispense medications, in conjunction with a physician or independently, to people with all kinds of health problems. Nurses work in a hospital, nursing home, doctor's office, clinic, and other facilities where health care is given.

A *registered nurse (RN)* is a health professional qualified to dispense medications, provide nursing care, and administer many complex treatments.

A *licensed practical nurse (LPN)* provides nursing care and gives treatments and medications under the supervision of a registered nurse.

Nurse practitioner. A nurse who specializes in a particular area of health care, such as mothers and children, families, or elderly people. Nurse practitioners may examine patients, make a diagnosis, and write prescriptions, usually while working closely with a doctor.

Nurse's aide. A health care worker who assists registered nurses and licensed practical nurses in providing health care in a hospital or other health care facility.

Obstetrician. A physician who delivers babies.

Occupational therapist. A health care professional who helps disabled people and others to regain, maintain, or improve their ability to manage ordinary living activities so they can live independently, or with minimal assistance. The occupa-

tional therapist often prescribes certain activities, such as arts and crafts.

Oncologist. A physician who treats people who have cancer.

Ophthalmologist. A physician who helps people to maintain healthy eyes and who treats eye diseases.

Optician. A health care professional who fills a doctor's prescription for eyeglasses.

Optometrist. A health care professional who tests vision and prescribes glasses.

Orthodontist. A dentist who repositions teeth to correct an inadequate bite, an unattractive appearance, or chewing difficulties.

Orthopedic surgeon. A physician who treats bone and joint diseases, often with surgery.

Otolaryngologist. *See* Ear, nose, and throat specialist.

Pathologist. A physician who specializes in the analysis of tissue samples and performs autopsies (dissections of dead persons' bodies) to detect diseases or to establish the cause of death.

Pediatrician. A physician who provides health care for healthy babies and children and treats them if they become ill.

Periodontist. A dentist who treats specific problems in tissues (gums) that surround the teeth.

Pharmacist. A health professional who prepares drugs prescribed by physicians, provides information about drugs, and sells health care products.

Physiatrist. A physician who helps people to regain strength and function in a limb or body part disabled by an injury, accident, or illness.

Physical therapist. A health professional trained to help disabled people regain muscle strength and mobility by using exercise, massage, and other treatments.

Physician's assistant (PA). A health professional trained to work under a physician's supervision in providing general health care and dispensing medications.

Plastic and reconstructive surgeon. A physician (surgeon) who specializes in performing surgical procedures for cosmetic reasons, or to correct body parts that are misshapen or do not function properly, from birth or due to injury, accident, or illness.

Podiatrist. A health professional who treats problems of the feet.

Psychiatrist. A physician who treats people with emotional or mental problems.

Psychologist. A specialist who studies mental functions and treats mental disorders.

Pulmonary disease specialist. A physician who specializes in diseases of the lungs, such as asthma or tuberculosis.

Radiation oncologist. A physician who prescribes and provides radiotherapy to treat certain diseases such as cancer.

Radiologist. A physician who uses X rays for diagnostic purposes.

Registered nurse (RN). *See* Nurse.

Social worker. A professional who works to help people with family, financial, and other problems.

Speech pathologist. A health professional trained to help people overcome speech problems.

Surgeon. A physician who performs operations to correct physical defects, remove abnormal growths, or treat illnesses caused by infection and other conditions.

Urologist. A physician who treats diseases of the genitourinary tract, or corrects defective organs and structures in this area.

D

Appendix E
BOOKS FOR TEENS

BOOKS FOR TEENS

Acne

Litt, Jerome. *Teen Skin from Head to Toe*. New York: Ballantine, 1986.

Novick, Nelson Lee. *Skin Care for Teens*. New York: Franklin Watts, 1988.

Silverstein, Alvin, et al. *Overcoming Acne: The How and Why of Healthy Skin Care*. New York: Morrow, 1990.

AIDS

Blake, Jeanne. *Risky Times: How to be AIDS Smart and Stay Healthy*. New York: Workman, 1990.

Hein, Karen, and Theresa Foy DiGeronimo. *AIDS: Trading Fears for Facts. A Guide for Young People*. Yonkers, NY: Consumer Reports Books, 1994.

Johnson, Earvin "Magic." *What You Can Do to Avoid AIDS*. New York: Times Books, 1995.

Landau, Elaine. *We Have AIDS*. New York: Franklin Watts, 1990.

Madaras, Lynda. *Lynda Madaras Talks to Teens About AIDS*. New York: Newmarket, 1988.

Nourse, Alan E., M.D. *Teen Guide to AIDS Prevention*. New York: Franklin Watts, 1990.

Alcoholism

See Substance Abuse

Allergies

Newman, Gerald, and Eleanor Newman Layfield. *Allergies*. New York: Franklin Watts, 1992.

Anxiety, Stress, Mental Illness

Buckingham, Robert, and Sandra Huggard. *Coping with Grief*. New York: Rosen, 1991.

Feldman, Robert S. *Understanding Stress*. New York: Franklin Watts, 1992.

Gilbert, Sara. *Get Help*. New York: Morrow, 1989.

Greenberg, Harvey. *Emotional Illness in Your Family: Helping Your Relative, Helping Yourself*. New York: Macmillan, 1989.

Maloney, Michael, and Rachel Kranz. *Straight Talk About Anxiety and Depression*. New York: Dell, 1993.

Newman, Susan. *Don't Be S.A.D.:A Teenage Guide to Handling Stress, Anxiety and Depression*. New York: Simon and Schuster, 1991.

Smith, Douglas W. *Schizophrenia*. New York: Franklin Watts, 1993.

Autoimmune Disease

Aaseng, Nathan. *Autoimmune Diseases*. New York: Franklin Watts, 1995.

Asthma

American Academy of Allergy, Asthma, and Immunology. *Managing Your Asthma*. (Free publication, call 800-456-2784).

Gershwin, M. E., and E. L. Klingelhofer. *Stop Suffering, Start Living*, 2nd ed. New York: Addison-Wesley, 1992.

Haas, F., M.D.; and S. S. Haas, M.D. *The Essential Asthma Book*. New York: Ivy Books, 1989.

Hyde, Margaret O., and Elizabeth H. Forsyth. *Living with Asthma*. New York: Walker, 1995.

Kerby, Mona. *Asthma*. New York: Franklin Watts, 1989.

Birth Control

See Family Planning/Contraception

Cancer

Bombeck, Erma. *I Want to Grow Hair, I Want to Grow Up, I Want to Go to Boise: Children Surviving Cancer*. New York: Harper, 1989.

Fine, Judylaine. *Afraid to Ask: A Book About Cancer*. New York: Lothrop, 1986.

Gravelle, Karen, and Bertram A. John. *Teenagers Face to Face with Cancer*. Englewood Cliffs: Messner, 1986.

Landau, Elaine. *Breast Cancer*. New York: Franklin Watts, 1995.

Cerebral Palsy

Aaseng, Nathan. *Cerebral Palsy*. New York: Franklin Watts, 1991.

Cystic Fibrosis

Silverstein, Alvin, et al. *Cystic Fibrosis*. New York: Franklin Watts, 1994.

Deafness and Hearing Loss

Mango, Karin. *Hearing Loss*. New York: Franklin Watts, 1991.

Depression and Suicide

Carter, Sharon, and Lawrence Clayton. *Coping with Depression*. New York: Rosen, 1990.

Hyde, Margaret O., and Elizabeth N. Forsyth. *Suicide*, 3rd ed. New York: Franklin Watts, 1991.

Silverstein, Herma. *Teenage Depression*. New York: Franklin Watts, 1990.

Diabetes

Goodheart, Barbara. *Diabetes*. New York: Franklin Watts, 1990.

Silverstein, Alvin et al. *Diabetes*. Hillside, NJ: Enslow, 1994.

Drug Abuse

See Substance Abuse

Eating Disorders and Dieting

Cauwels, Janice M. *Bulimia*. New York: Doubleday, 1985.

Kolodny, Jancy J. *When Food's a Foe: How to Confront and Conquer Eating Disorders*, rev. ed. Boston: Little, Brown, 1992.

Landau, Elaine. *Weight: A Teenage Concern*. New York: Dutton/Lodestar, 1991.

McMillan, Daniel. *Obesity*. New York: Franklin Watts, 1994.

Sonder, Ben. *Eating Disorders: When Food Turns Against You*. New York: Franklin Watts, 1993.

Thayne, Emma Lou, and Becky Thayne Markosian. *Hope and Recovery: A Mother-Daughter Story About Anorexia Nervosa, Bulimia, and Manic Depression*. New York: Franklin Watts, 1992.

Wardell, Judy. *Thin Within*. New York: Harmony Books, 1991.

Family Planning/Contraception

Benson, Michael. *Coping with Birth Control*, rev. ed. New York: Rosen, 1992.

Freeman, Sarah, and Vern Bullough. *The Complete Guide to Fertility and Family Planning*. New York: Prometheus Books, 1992.

Nourse, Alan E., M.D. *Teen Guide to Birth Control*. New York: Franklin Watts, 1988.

Planned Parenthood Association. *A Family Planning Library Manual*, 5th ed. New York: Planned Parenthood, 1994.

Winikoff, Beverly, Suzanne Wymelenberg, and the editors. *The Contraceptive Handbook: A Guide to Safe and Effective Choices*. Yonkers, NY: Consumer Reports Books, 1992.

Feelings and Relationships

Bolick, Nancy O'Keefe. *How to Survive Your Parents' Divorce*. New York: Franklin Watts, 1994.

Booher, Dianna. *Coping: When Your Family Falls Apart*. New York: Julian Messner, 1991.

Gardner, Richard. *The Boys' and Girls' Book About Divorce*. New York: Bantam, 1992.

Rofes, Eric, ed. *The Kids' Book of Divorce: By, For, and About Kids*. New York: Vintage Books, 1982.

E

Vedral, Joyce. *I Can't Take It Anymore*. New York: Ballantine Books, 1987.

———. *My Parents Are Driving Me Crazy*. New York: Ballantine Books, 1992.

Weston, Carol. *Girltalk*. New York: Harper Perennial, 1992.

Wolf, Anthony. *Get Out of My Life . . . But First, Could You Drive Me and Cheryl to the Mall?* New York: Noonday, 1991.

Gay and Lesbian Concerns

Brimner, Larry Dane. *Being Different: Lambda Youths Speak Out*. New York: Franklin Watts, 1995.

Cohen, Susan, and Daniel Cohen. *When Someone You Know Is Gay*. New York: Evans, 1989.

Heron, Ann, ed. *One Teenager in Ten: Writings by Gay and Lesbian Youth*. Boston: Alyson, 1983.

Pollack, Rachel, and Cheryl Schwartz. *The Journey Out: A Guide for and About Lesbian, Gay, and Bisexual Teens*. New York: Viking, 1995.

Rench, Janice E. *Understanding Sexual Identity: A Book for Gay Teens and Their Friends*. Minneapolis: Lerner, 1990.

Heart Disease

Arnold, Caroline. *Heart Disease*. New York: Franklin Watts, 1990.

Hepatitis

Silverstein, Alvin, et al. *Hepatitis*. Hillside, NJ: Enslow, 1994.

Learning Disabilities

Levine, Mel. *Keeping a Head in School: A Student's Book About Learning Disabilities and Learning Disorders*. Cambridge: Educators Publishing Service, 1990.

Savage, John F. *Dyslexia: Understanding Reading Problems*. Englewood Cliffs: Julian Messner, 1985.

Leukemia

Siegel, Dorothy S., and David E. Newton. *Leukemia*. New York: Franklin Watts, 1994.

Mononucleosis

Silverstein, Alvin, et al. *Mononucleosis*. Hillside, NJ: Enslow, 1994.

Muscular Dystrophy

Corrick, James A. *Muscular Dystrophy*. New York: Franklin Watts, 1992.

Physical Disabilities

Krementz, Jill. *How It Feels to Live with a Physical Disability*. New York: Simon and Schuster, 1992.

Kriegsman, Kay Harris, Elinor L. Zaslow, and Jennifer D'Zmura-Rechsteiner. *Taking Charge: Teenagers Talk About Life and Physical Disabilities*. Rockville, MD: Woodbine House, 1992.

Physical Fitness

Micheli, Lyle. *Sportsense for the Young Athlete: A Parent's Guide to Fun and Safe Fitness*. New York: Houghton Mifflin, 1990.

Simon, Nissa. *Good Sports*. New York: HarperCollins, 1990.

Pregnancy and Parenting

Bode, Janet. *Kids Still Having Kids: People Talk About Teen Pregnancy*. New York: Franklin Watts, 1992.

Hawksley, Jane. *Teen Guide to Pregnancy, Drugs, and Smoking*. New York: Franklin Watts, 1989.

Kitzinger, Sheila. *The Complete Book of Pregnancy and Childbirth*, rev. ed. New York: Knopf, 1989.

Kuklin, Susan. *What Do I Do Now? Talking About Teenage Pregnancy*. New York: Putnam, 1991.

Lang, Paul, and Susan Lang. *Teen Fathers*. New York: Franklin Watts, 1995.

Silverstein, Herma. *Teen Guide to Single Parenting*. New York: Franklin Watts, 1989.

Puberty

Bell, Alison, and Lisa Rooney. *Your Body,*

Yourself. Chicago: Contemporary Books, 1993.

Bell, Ruth, et al. *Chaging Bodies, Changing Lives*, rev. ed. New York: Random House, 1988.

Madaras, Lynda, and Dane Saavedra. *The What's Happening to My Body? Book for Boys: A Growing up Guide for Parents and Sons*, rev. ed. New York: Newmarket, 1993.

Madaras, Lynda, and Area Madaras. *The What's Happening to My Body? Book for Girls: A Growing up Guide for Parents and Daughters*, rev. ed. New York: Newmarket, 1993.

McCoy, Kathy, and Charles Wibbelsman. *The New Teenage Body Book*. New York: Putnam, 1992.

Packer, Kenneth L. *Puberty: The Story of Growth and Change*. New York: Franklin Watts, 1989.

Rape

See Sexual Abuse and Assault

Sex

Boston Children's Hospital. *What Teenagers Want to Know About Sex: Questions and Answers*. Boston: Little, Brown, 1988.

Gordon, Sol. *Facts About Sex for Teenage Youth*. Glendale, CA: Prometheus, 1992.

Johnson, Eric W. *Love and Sex in Plain Language*, rev. ed. New York: Bantam, 1988.

Nourse, Alan E., M.D. *Teen Guide to Safe Sex*. New York: Franklin Watts, 1988.

Pomeroy, Wardell. *Girls and Sex*. New York: Delacorte, 1991.

———. *Boys and Sex*. New York: Dell, 1993.

Terkel, Susan Neiburg. *Finding Your Way: A Book About Sexual Ethics*. New York: Franklin Watts, 1995.

Warren, Andrea, and Jay Wiedenkeller. *Everybody's Doing It*. New York: Penguin, 1993.

Westheimer, Ruth, and Nathan Kravetz. *First Love: A Young People's Guide to Sexual Information*. New York: Warner, 1986.

Sexual Abuse and Assault

Benedict, Helen. *Safe, Strong, and Streetwise*. Boston: Little, Brown, 1987.

Bode, Janet. *The Voices of Rape*. New York: Franklin Watts, 1990.

Booher, Dianna D. *Rape, What Would You Do If?* rev. ed. New York: Julian Messner, 1991.

Dolan, Edward F. *Child Abuse*, rev. ed. New York: Franklin Watts, 1992.

Kosof, Anna. *Battered Women: Living with the Enemy*. New York: Franklin Watts, 1995.

———. *Incest: Families in Crisis*. New York: Franklin Watts, 1985.

Mufson, Susan, and Rachel Kranz. *Straight Talk About Child Abuse*. New York: Facts on File, 1991.

Parrot, Andrea. *Coping with Date Rape and Acquaintance Rape*. New York: Rosen, 1988.

Rue, Nancy N. *Coping with Dating Violence*. New York: Rosen, 1989.

Sexually Transmitted Diseases

Daugirdas. John T., M.D. *STD: Sexually Transmitted Diseases, Including HIV/AIDS*. Hinsdale, IL: Medtext, 1992.

Little, Marjorie. *Sexually Transmitted Diseases*. New York: Chelsea House, 1991.

Nourse, Alan E., M. D. *Sexually Transmitted Diseases*. New York: Franklin Watts, 1992.

Sickle Cell Anemia

Beshore, George. *Sickle Cell Anemia*. New York: Franklin Watts, 1994.

Steroids

Lukas, Scott. *Steroids*. Hillside, NJ: Enslow, 1994.

Nuwer, Hank. *Steroids*. New York: Franklin Watts, 1990.

Substance Abuse

Berger, Gilda. *Addiction*, rev. ed. New York: Franklin Watts, 1992.

———. *Alcoholism and the Family*. New York: Franklin Watts, 1993.

Berger, Gilda, and Nancy Levitin. *Crack: The*

E

New Drug Epidemic, rev. ed. New York: Franklin Watts, 1994.

Claypool, Jane. *Alcohol and You*, rev. ed. New York: Franklin Watts, 1988.

Dolan, Edward F. *Drugs in Sports*, rev. ed. New York: Franklin Watts, 1992.

McMillan, Daniel. *Winning the Battle Against Drugs: Rehabilitation Programs*. New York: Franklin Watts, 1991.

Ryan, Elizabeth A. *Straight Talk About Drugs and Alcohol*. New York: Dell, 1992.

Toma, David, and Chris Biffle. *Drugs: Turning Your Life Around*. New York: Harper Perennial, 1992.

Yoslow, Mark. *Drugs in the Body: Effects of Abuse*. New York: Franklin Watts, 1992.

Suicide *See* Depression and Suicide

Tuberculosis

Landau, Elaine. *Tuberculosis*. New York: Franklin Watts, 1995.

Silverstein, Alvin, et al. *Tuberculosis*. Hillside, NJ: Enslow, 1994.

Viruses

Nourse, Alan E., M.D. *The Virus Invaders*. New York: Franklin Watts, 1992.

BOOKS FOR PARENTS

Bain, Lisa J., for the Children's Hospital of Philadelphia. *A Parent's Guide to Attention Deficit Disorders*. New York: Delta, 1991.

Fairchild, Betty, and Nancy Hayward. *Now That You Know: What Every Parent Should Know About Homosexuality*. San Diego: Harcourt Brace Jovanovich, 1979.

Jablow, Martha M., for the Children's Hospital of Philadelphia. *A Parent's Guide to Eating Disorders and Obesity*. New York: Delta, 1992.

Klagsbrun, Frances. *To Die Too Young: Youth and Suicide*. Boston: Houghton Mifflin, 1976.

Narramore, Bruce, M.D.; and Vern Lewis, M.D. *Parenting Teens: A Road Map Through the Ages and Stages of Adolescence*. Wheaton, IL: Tyndale House, 1990.

Oster, Gerald, M.D.; and Sarah Montgomery, M.S.W. *Helping Your Depressed Teenager: A Guide for Parents and Caregivers*. New York: John Wiley & Sons, 1995.

Phelan, Thomas. *Surviving Your Adolescents: How to Manage and Let Go of Your 13–16 Year Olds*. Glen Ellyn, IL: Child Management, 1993.

Powell, Douglas N. Teenagers: *When to Worry and What to Do*. New York: Doubleday, 1986.

Steinberg, Laurence, and Ann Levine. *You and Your Adolescent*. New York: Harper & Row, 1990.

E

Appendix F

FIRST AID

First Aid consists of urgent care, in emergency situations. This involves care given after an automobile accident, sports emergency, or any sudden injury or illness that creates a serious threat to the victim's health and, possibly, life. The victim's survival may depend on the First Aid measures provided by someone at the scene, until medical help arrives and provides safe transport and hospital care for the victim.

The American Red Cross (ARC), and other health care organizations—for example, a local ambulance corps—offer courses in First Aid, Basic Life Support (BLS), and Advanced Life Support (ALS). Call the ARC (check your local telephone directory, or ask the operator) for information about nearby courses. On successful completion of a First Aid course, you will be certified as a First Aid provider. The information here provides an overview of First Aid measures to use in an emergency until medical help arrives. Remember: This is *not* a First Aid course. A formal First Aid course consists of a period of formal instruction with hands-on practice, under the supervision of a qualified First Aid instructor.

The term First Aid is also used for the basic treatment given for minor injuries. This involves simple household treatment measures such as an ice bag for a swelling caused by an insect bite, or antiseptic solution and a sterile (Band-aid) dressing applied to a cut. For all but minor emergencies, always call, or have someone else call, 911 or the local emergency assistance number, to quickly obtain medical help and professional emergency care for the victim.

F

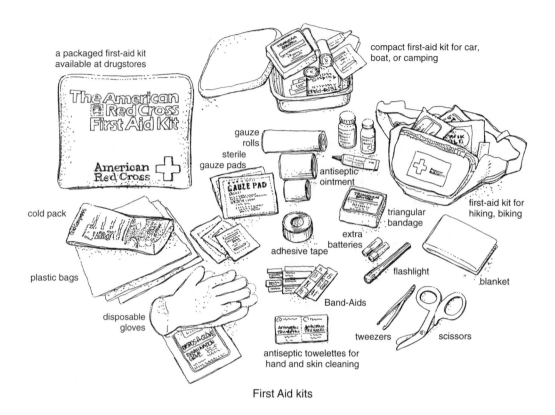

a packaged first-aid kit available at drugstores

compact first-aid kit for car, boat, or camping

gauze rolls

sterile gauze pads

antiseptic ointment

cold pack

first-aid kit for hiking, biking

triangular bandage

extra batteries

adhesive tape

plastic bags

flashlight

blanket

disposable gloves

Band-Aids

tweezers

scissors

antiseptic towelettes for hand and skin cleaning

First Aid kits

COMMON EMERGENCIES—IMMEDIATE FIRST AID MEASURES

If you have to handle an emergency situation with an injured person, follow these steps:

- Call 911 or other local emergency service.
- Check for a Medic-Alert bracelet or pendant. These are worn by people with specific conditions and diseases (examples are diabetes, epilepsy, severe allergy) that may require specialized assistance. Follow the instructions inscribed on the Medic-Alert.
- Follow the ABCs OF FIRST AID. Confusion may delay life-saving efforts in an emergency. To avoid this, keep in mind the ABCs of emergency care for a seriously injured person.

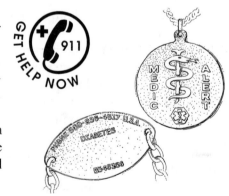

A – Airway. A person must have open, functioning air passages (respiratory tract) to be able to breathe. These passages include the nose, mouth, throat, bronchi, and lungs. If a person cannot breathe, you must quickly find the reason, then act to restore respirations. *See* A person is not breathing, Artificial respiration (mouth-to-mouth resuscitation); A person is choking, Heimlich maneuver. *Inability to breathe is a life-threatening emergency.*

F

B – Bleeding. If a person is bleeding profusely from a major blood vessel, such as an artery, First Aid measures must be used promptly to stop the bleeding or the victim will die. *See* A person is bleeding heavily. *Heavy bleeding (hemorrhage) is a life-threatening emergency.*

C – cardiopulmonary resuscitation – CPR. CPR must be administered promptly for a person in cardiac arrest (the heart has stopped beating, and the victim is not breathing). If the heart and respirations are not restarted within five minutes, the victim will suffer permanent brain damage due to oxy-

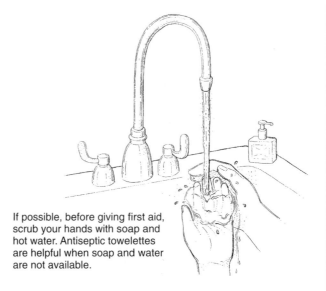

If possible, before giving first aid, scrub your hands with soap and hot water. Antiseptic towelettes are helpful when soap and water are not available.

gen deprivation. If more time elapses, the victim will die. *See* A person is not breathing, Cardiac arrest. *A stopped heart and respirations are life-threatening emergencies.*

The sections below tell how to assess a victim, and what to do while waiting for medical assistance. The First Aid section also describes other situations that are not life-threatening but may involve pain, discomfort, infection, and other serious complications.

A PERSON IS NOT BREATHING—A major emergency—Call 911!

Breathing (respiration) is essential to life. Breathing may stop for many different reasons: loss of consciousness, which may cause the tongue to slide down the back of the throat and block the airway, or mucus secretions or other objects that block air from reaching the lungs. Other causes include drowning, being subjected to chemical or other toxic fumes, a heart attack, or contact with a strong electric current. *See* Cardiac arrest and CPR; A person is choking, Heimlich maneuver.

WHAT YOU CAN DO
Give artificial (mouth-to-mouth) respiration
- Call 911 or your local emergency number.
- Test to be certain that the person has actually stopped breathing: if the victim's face has an unhealthy, blue-gray color, if the victim is not exhaling any air (hold your fingers in front of the mouth to test), and if the chest and abdomen do not rise and fall, he or she is not breathing.
  Note: A victim of electric shock must be removed from the source of current *before* being given First Aid. *See* Electric shock.

F

- Clear the airway: Run a finger through the victim's mouth and upper throat to remove any obstruction.
- Start artificial respiration (mouth-to-mouth resuscitation):

If the victim is not breathing, but has a pulse, lay the victim on his or her back, turn the head to one side, remove any debris (fluid, mucus, vomit) from the mouth, tilt back the head, and pull up the chin.

Place your mouth over the victim's mouth, close (pinch) the nostrils closed with your fingers, and blow into the victim's mouth with enough force to make his or her chest rise, about 14 times per minute.

If the victim is a small child, don't tilt the head back as far as you would an adult's, to prevent cutting off the airway. Blow gently, while covering the child's nose and mouth with your mouth, about 15 breaths per minute for a small child, 20 breaths per minute for an infant.

After each breath into the victim's mouth, wait for him or her to breathe out (exhale), then continue giving artificial respiration.

If the victim does not exhale (the chest and abdomen do not rise and fall), look inside the mouth to see if the tongue has slipped back, blocking the air passages. In that case, pull the tongue out of the way and repeat your blowing efforts until breathing starts or medical help arrives.

If the victim does not start breathing after several minutes, an obstruction may be present somewhere in the throat, requiring performance of the Heimlich maneuver. *See* A person is choking, Heimlich maneuver.

Mouth-to-mouth resuscitation (rescue breathing)

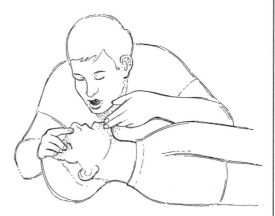

1. Tilt the person's head back and lift the chin

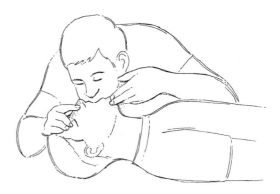

2. Pinch the nose shut. Place your mouth over the person's and give two full breaths. Then give about twelve more breaths, for a total of 14 a minute.

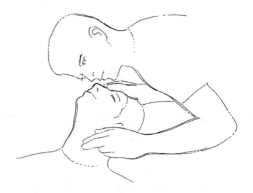

3. Check for a pulse. If pulse is present, continue rescue breathing until help arrives or person begins breathing. If no pulse, begin CPR.

A PERSON IS CHOKING—A life-threatening emergency—Call 911!

Choking occurs when a piece of food or a small object placed in the mouth slips into the throat and obstructs the airway. If the person can still breathe, he or she may be able to cough up the blockage. If the person is unable to breathe, and cannot cough up the food or object stuck in the throat, emergency assistance is essential.

+☎ 911 GET HELP NOW

WHAT YOU CAN DO

- You don't need to do anything immediately as long as the person or child keeps coughing, the color of the face is healthy, and they remain conscious.
- Carefully observe the victim until the food or other object is coughed up, and the person is breathing normally. If it is not dislodged, get medical help.
- IF THE VICTIM TURNS BLUE, CANNOT SPEAK, CLUTCHES THE THROAT, OR BECOMES UNCONSCIOUS: PERFORM THE HEIMLICH MANEUVER.
  This is the procedure:

1. Stand behind the choking person, and wrap your arms around the waist and the bottom of the victim's rib cage.
2. Grab your right fist with your left hand, then push in and upward on the victim's upper abdomen with a sudden thrusting motion, as forceful as possible. This action pushes the food up and out through the victim's mouth, and prevents asphyxiation.

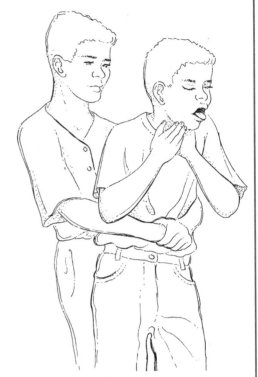
Using the Heimlich maneuver

IF A SMALL CHILD IS CHOKING

- Sit down and place the child face down, legs toward you, across one knee.
- Give a few gentle thumps on the child's upper back, between the shoulder blades. **Caution:** Thump a little child much more gently than you would an adult. For an infant, place one hand under the chest, and thump the baby's back with your other hand.
- Continue thumping gently until the piece of food or other object is coughed up, or medical help arrives.

IF THE CHOKING PERSON IS UNCONSCIOUS

1. Perform the Heimlich maneuver.
2. Lay the victim flat on his or her back.
3. Kneel, straddling the victim below the hips.
4. Place your hands, one on top of the other, on the victim's abdomen below the breast-

F

bone. Press sharply upward toward the chest with the heel of your bottom hand, to expel the material that caused the choking.

5. Turn the victim's head to one side to remove material.
6. Repeat the above steps if food or other material is not dislodged and expelled after the first effort.

A PERSON IS BLEEDING HEAVILY—A major emergency—Call 911!

Heavy blood loss (hemorrhage)—a loss of more than one or two pints —may cause shock, loss of consciousness, and death if not quickly stopped. Life-threatening bleeding in healthy people is most often caused by a serious injury or accident, in which a large blood vessel is severed.

WHAT YOU CAN DO

- Have the victim lie flat, to prevent fainting and further injury.
- Use a sterile piece of gauze dressing, if handy. If not, place a clean cloth or rag over the wound and apply steady pressure. Add more gauze or clean dressings on top of saturated dressings if blood soaks through. Don't lift the dressings to see if bleeding has stopped.
- Elevate the body part to help control bleeding, if possible.
- Apply pressure above the wound, on an arterial pressure point, if direct pressure does not stop the bleeding.

    If these measures don't work, and the wound is deep, in an arm or leg: press hard with one or two fingers, or with your hand on the artery above the wound, on the inner part of the upper arm, or the inner part of the thigh, just below the groin. *See illustration* Arterial Pressure points, page 175.

    Note: Do not try to apply pressure on an artery if the victim is bleeding from the head, neck, or trunk.

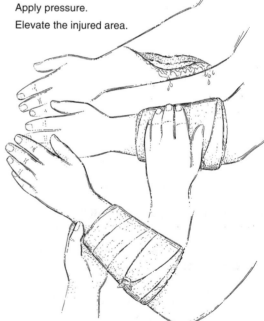

A wound with heavy bleeding

Control the bleeding by placing a clean dressing or cloth over the wound. Wrap a bandage or strip of cloth over the dressing.

Apply pressure.

Elevate the injured area.

- Use a tourniquet only as a last resort, if the above measures fail to control the bleeding. Never use a tourniquet in the area of the head, neck, or trunk.

    Caution: A tourniquet may cut circulation and lead to the loss of a limb.

    To apply a tourniquet, cut a strip of cloth several inches wide, and long enough to go around the limb at least twice. Wrap the strip tightly, without touching the wound,

174

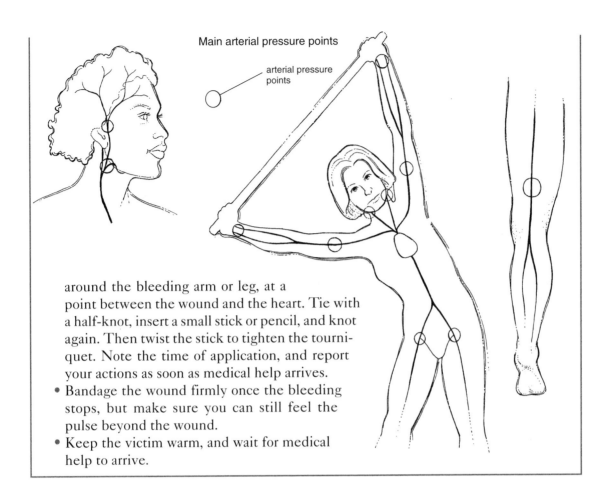

Main arterial pressure points

arterial pressure points

around the bleeding arm or leg, at a point between the wound and the heart. Tie with a half-knot, insert a small stick or pencil, and knot again. Then twist the stick to tighten the tourniquet. Note the time of application, and report your actions as soon as medical help arrives.

- Bandage the wound firmly once the bleeding stops, but make sure you can still feel the pulse beyond the wound.
- Keep the victim warm, and wait for medical help to arrive.

CARDIAC ARREST (THE HEART STOPS)—A major emergency—Call 911!

When a person's heart stops, breathing stops too, along with other body functions. The heart may stop beating after a heart attack, or due to other heart conditions, or after major trauma or injury. The victim will suffer irreversible brain damage (due to lack of blood reaching the brain and other body parts) if not resuscitated within a few minutes. If more time elapses, death is inevitable.

GET HELP NOW 911

CPR—cardio- (heart), pulmonary (lungs) resuscitation (rescue)—can save the life of a person in cardiac arrest. CPR can be administered by one or by two trained First Aiders. Preferably, two trained persons should perform CPR.

WHAT YOU CAN DO
Give CPR—one First Aider

- Clear the victim's airway. *See* A person is not breathing.
- Check for breathing and pulse at the wrist or neck. *See* A person is not breathing.

If the victim is not breathing and has no pulse

1. Lay the victim flat on his or her back on a firm surface.

F

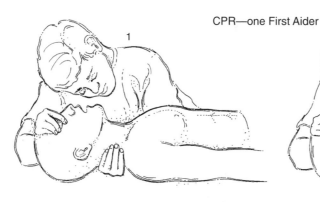
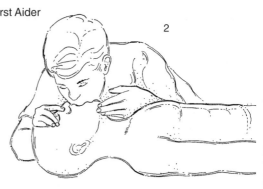

2. Tilt the victim's head back so the chin is elevated, take a deep breath, and give the victim 4 to 6 deep mouth-to-mouth breaths.

3. Place the heel of your right hand on the lower tip of the victim's breastbone, and your left hand on top of your right hand.

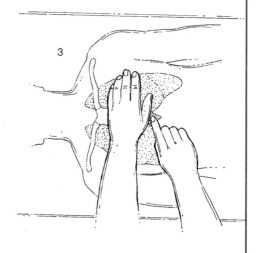

4. Depress the victim's breastbone firmly and forcefully about 1^1/$_2$" to 2", then release the pressure.

5. Continue the pattern of 15 chest compressions, followed by two mouth-to-mouth breaths, to add up to 60 to 80 chest compressions and 10 mouth-to-mouth breaths per minute. Squeeze down hard on the chest to force the heart to pump blood through the body, and blow air into the lungs, until the

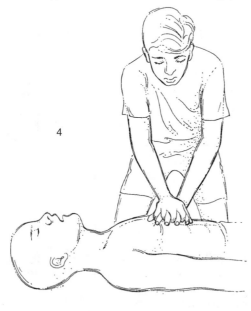
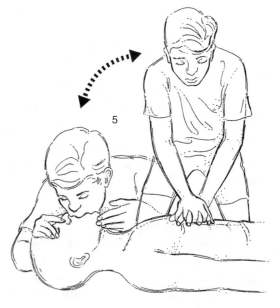

F

victim has a pulse and is breathing, or medical help arrives. (Stop CPR for no more than five seconds while you check the victim's pulse and breathing.)

Give CPR—two First Aiders

- First Aider I kneels next to the victim's head and gives one mouth-to-mouth breath to each five chest compressions performed by First Aider II—at a rate of 12 to 16 breaths per minute given by First Aider I, to 60 to 80 chest compressions per minute given by First Aider II. (If the victim is a small child, use a rate of two breaths for every five chest compressions.)
- Continue CPR until the victim regains a pulse and starts breathing unassisted or until medical help arrives.

AN UNCONSCIOUS PERSON—A major emergency—Call 911!

A person may lose consciousness as a result of a blow, accident, other injury, or illness.

WHAT YOU CAN DO

- Check to see if the victim is breathing. If not, remove any obstruction in the airway, and start artificial respiration (mouth-to-mouth resuscitation). *See* A person is not breathing.
- Check the victim's pulse. If there is no pulse, the victim's heart has stopped beating. Perform CPR. *See* Cardiac arrest, CPR.
- Once breathing and a heartbeat are restored, turn the victim onto one side, the head and chin forward and lower than the body.
- Keep the victim warm with clothing or blankets.
- Check the victim's breathing and pulse frequently.
- Stay with the victim until medical help arrives.

A PERSON HAS BEEN BURNED

Burns can be caused by heat, flames, or contact with boiling hot water. Other burns may be caused by contact with chemical substances or gases.

First-degree scald or burn—Can be treated without medical assistance. Only superficial layers of skin are involved; skin may be red, without blisters.

Second-degree burn—Call 911: Requires medical follow-up. All but the deepest layer of the skin are harmed. The skin may or may not blister.

Third-degree burn—A Major Emergency—Call 911! All skin layers and possibly tissues under the skin are involved. Appearance of the skin may be white or black, and scarred.

WHAT YOU CAN DO

For a first-degree burn (minor scald or burn)

- Plunge burned part into cold water. If unable to immerse, apply cold compresses, using clean sheets or towels. Apply cold until pain stops.

F

- If burn continues to cause pain, shows signs of infection, or starts to blister, obtain medical help.

For second- and third-degree burns (severe scald or burn). Call 911!
- Pour water on burning area (hair, clothing), if flames are still present.
- Use a coat or blanket to smother fire elsewhere on body.
- Cut clothes away from burned area and remove, unless they stick.
- Wash your hands, then apply thick, sterile dressings or clean sheets or towels, to relieve pain and keep area clean.
- If the victim is in shock, give First Aid for shock. *See* A person in shock.

A PERSON HAS A CHEMICAL BURN—A major emergency—Call 911!

Chemical burns are caused by skin contact with a strong acid or alkaline substance such as phenol, phosphorus, and other substances frequently used in industry.

WHAT YOU CAN DO
- Flush the affected area with water for several minutes, to wash off or dilute the chemical substance.
- If the substance has affected the eyes, flush the eyes with water, pouring it toward the outer portion of the face, then cover the eyes with a clean or sterile dressing until medical help arrives.

A PERSON IS DROWNING—A major emergency—Call 911!

A drowning person's chances of survival depend on how long he or she has been submerged, the temperature of the water, and the breathing or other problems caused by water in the respiratory (air passages) tract and gastrointestinal (gullet, stomach, intestines) tract.

WHAT YOU CAN DO
Give artificial respiration; cardiopulmonary resuscitation (CPR)
- Start artificial respiration as quickly as possible, even while pulling the victim from the water.
- Get the victim out of the water. With the victim on his or her back, turn the head to one side so fluids can drain from the mouth.
- Check the victim's pulse and breathing.
- If the victim does not breathe and has no pulse: give mouth-to-mouth breathing, or CPR, as needed, until the heart starts beating and the victim is breathing.
- Keep the victim warm.
- Get the victim to a hospital emergency room as quickly as possible for further treatment and observation.

F

A PERSON IN SHOCK—A major emergency—Call 911!

Shock is a reaction by the body to a severe trauma, such as a burn or great loss of blood. It must be treated promptly to prevent circulatory failure. Symptoms include weakness; pale, cold, moist skin; irregular, shallow breathing; rapid pulse; nausea; low blood pressure; and insufficient production of urine. Shock may not develop until later (delayed shock).

WHAT YOU CAN DO

- Have the person lie down, and lower the head to a level below the feet—provided there is no head or chest injury.
- Control bleeding. *See* A person is bleeding heavily.
- Loosen clothing to ease breathing.
- Keep the person warm with clothing or blankets.
- Wait for the ambulance.

A PERSON HAS RECEIVED AN ELECTRIC SHOCK—A major emergency—Call 911!

Contact with a strong electric current can cause severe burns, stoppage of breathing and the heart (cardiac arrest), and death. Never touch a victim of electric shock until the current has been turned off or the victim separated from the source of the current.

WHAT YOU CAN DO
First: Break contact with the current

- If outdoors: Call the police, fire department, or electric company to disconnect the current.
  While waiting, you may be able to break victim contact with a high-tension wire or cable by using a branch, or wooden pole, or other nonmetallic device (that does not conduct electricity) to push the victim away from the source of the current, the live wire, or other current-carrying device.
- If indoors: Turn off the current by disconnecting the appliance, or through the switch of the fuse box, to separate the victim from live current.
  Note: A person struck by lightning does not conduct electricity and can therefore receive immediate First Aid.

WHAT TO DO NEXT FOR THE ELECTRIC SHOCK VICTIM

- Check respirations (breathing), and pulse.
- Clear the airway; provide artificial respiration (mouth-to-mouth resuscitation) or CPR, if the victim is in cardiac arrest. *See* A person who is not breathing, cardiac arrest.
- Treat any burn. *See* A person has been burned.
- Take victim to the hospital as quickly as possible.

F

A PERSON HAS BEEN RAPED

Sexual assault and rape are major problems during adolescence, as at other periods of life. Males as well as females may be victimized. Prompt medical attention, counseling, and support may help the victim's recovery and perhaps reduce the long-term damage.

WHAT YOU CAN DO

- If the victim needs immediate First Aid, refer to the First Aid section for treatment of the specific injury.

  - If the person is unconscious, *see* A person is not breathing, An unconscious person.
  - If the person is bleeding, *see* A person is bleeding heavily, A person with cuts or scrapes.
  - If the person has broken bones or a spinal injury, *see* A person has a fracture, A person may have a broken neck or back injury.
  - If the person is in shock, *see* A person in shock.

- To help authorities identify the attacker, instruct the rape victim not to change clothing, shower, or brush his or her teeth.
- Provide comfort, in person or by telephone.
- Report the crime to the police.
- Encourage the victim to call a rape hotline, or place the call yourself.
- Encourage the person to seek medical attention at an emergency room, clinic, or medical office.
- Accompany the person to the emergency room, or arrange for a friend or family member to do this.

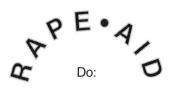

RAPE • AID

Do:

- Restore breathing and circulation
- Stop the bleeding
- Treat broken bones
- Treat for shock
- Provide comfort
- Call the police
- Call for assistance
- Call a doctor

Don't Allow Victim

- to change clothes
- take a shower
- brush teeth

IN THE EMERGENCY ROOM

- Many hospitals have a rape counselor on call. This person will help the victim deal with the medical staff, police, and others.
- A complete physical exam is performed. Samples of body fluids, hair, fingernail scrapings, and blood are collected and sent to a lab for analysis. Clothing is also sent for analysis.
- Female victims are given a pregnancy test if necessary.
- Postcoital contraception (morning-after pill) is offered.
- Antibiotics are provided to prevent chlamydial infection, gonorrhea, and syphilis.
- The patient is offered a follow-up medical visit and HIV counseling and testing.
- The police interview the victim and begin the investigation of the crime.
- Unless physical injuries require hospitalization, the victim may be released, usually with an appointment for follow-up counseling.

F

A PERSON HAS HEATSTROKE OR SUNSTROKE—A major emergency—Call 911!

Sunstroke or heatstroke may develop after long exposure to hot sun, or high temperatures. The body may become unable to get rid of stored-up heat. Symptoms are: high body temperature (up to 106°F.), absence of perspiration, dry skin, dehydration, headache, numbness, rapid pulse and breathing, confusion, and coma (which may lead to death if treatment is not provided quickly).

WHAT YOU CAN DO
- Remove the person from the sun and have him or her lie down in a cool, shady place.
- Remove the person's outer clothes.
- Sponge the person with cool water.
- If a fan is available, direct it at the person's body.
- Send the person to the hospital for further treatment.

A PERSON HAS A FRACTURE (BROKEN BONE)—Not life-threatening, but requires medical help—Call 911!

There are different types of fractures; First Aid depends on the type of fracture sustained by the victim: a simple (closed) fracture is a simple break in a bone; other tissues in the area are intact. Or you may find a comminuted (open, compound) fracture—a bone break in one or several places, with an open wound above the point of break.

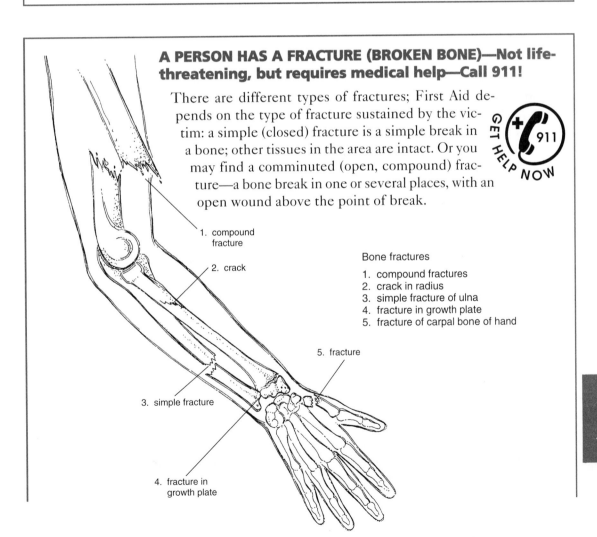

1. compound fracture
2. crack
5. fracture
3. simple fracture
4. fracture in growth plate

Bone fractures

1. compound fractures
2. crack in radius
3. simple fracture of ulna
4. fracture in growth plate
5. fracture of carpal bone of hand

F

WHAT YOU CAN DO
For a simple fracture

Have victim lie down comfortably. Do not try to set the bone. If medical help is not immediately available:

- Use one or two splints (boards, broomsticks, or splints made with rolled-up newspapers, long enough to reach from above to below the break), and pad them with a sheet, towel, or other material.
- Place either one splint next to the break, or a splint on each side of the broken bone, without changing the shape of the limb as you find it.
- Use bandages or strips of sheeting to keep the splint(s) in place. Do not fasten the bandages or strips too tightly: only enough to immobilize the limb during the trip to the emergency room.
- Apply an ice bag—if available—to the painful area.

For a comminuted fracture

- Do not try to push the bone back in place.
- Use splints, as for a simple fracture, above, to immobilize the area of the break(s).

A PERSON MAY HAVE A BROKEN NECK OR BACK (SPINAL INJURY)— A major emergency—Call 911!

Suspect a broken neck if: the victim says the shoulder area feels numb, is tingling, or the fingers do not move readily. Suspect a broken back if: the victim is able to move the fingers, but not the feet or toes, or feels tingling or numbness in those areas.

WHAT YOU CAN DO

- Don't try to move or lift the victim's head.
- Loosen the victim's clothing, and keep the victim from moving.
- If you must move the victim, try to find a firm board or other rigid support, such as a door or ironing board.
- Keeping the victim's body in a straight line, place him or her on the board before attempting a move.

A PERSON HAS A SEIZURE (CONVULSION)

There are two types of seizures:

Petit mal seizures. A person who has a petit mal seizure may have a loss of consciousness for several seconds. No treatment is usually needed for this type of seizure.

Grand mal seizures. A person who has a grand mal seizure may lose consciousness for up to several minutes, while the body shakes and thrashes uncontrollably.

WHAT YOU CAN DO
For a grand mal seizure: call 911—victim needs a medical evaluation

- Lay the person gently on the floor.
- Turn the head to one side, to prevent choking.
- Remove nearby furniture or other objects to prevent injury.
- Never place your fingers in the victim's mouth: the teeth may clamp down and injure you.
- Once the seizure ends, let the person rest for a while. He or she may be temporarily confused, and unable to remember the seizure.
- If breathing difficulties develop after a prolonged seizure, give artificial (mouth-to-mouth) respiration until medical help arrives.

A CASE OF POISONING—Any kind of poisoning is a major emergency— Call 911!

There are many different causes of poisoning.

Household poisons or other chemical poisons
A small child may ingest a common household cleaner, such as ammonia, bleach, detergent, or drain cleaner (and many others), or swallow the contents of a bottle of prescription or over-the-counter drugs. An adult may ingest a chemical agent by accident, or intentionally, in an attempt to commit suicide. Poisoning can also result after inhaling poisonous smoke, gas, or chemical fumes.

WHAT YOU CAN DO
Household poisons
- Look for the source of the poisoning, and check the label.
- Give the recommended antidote, call for an ambulance, or take the victim to a hospital emergency room.
- While waiting for help, contact the nearest Poison Control Center. Check your telephone directory under "Emergency listings," or ask the telephone operator for the listing.
- Describe the product to the Poison Control Center, and take it or the label with you to the hospital.

Poisonous smoke, gas, or chemical fumes
- Don't try to rescue the victim yourself when the source of poisoning is smoke, gas, or chemical fumes. Call experienced rescuers, such as police or firefighters.
- If no help is immediately available, take a few deep breaths, inhale, and hold your breath when you enter the contaminated area. Stay close to the ground so you won't inhale the rising fumes. As quickly as possible, pull the person out into the fresh air.
- Give artificial respiration (mouth-to-mouth resuscitation) if the person has stopped breathing, and loosen the victim's clothing.

F

- Seek medical help as quickly as possible, even if the victim recovers and feels much better.

Carbon monoxide (CO) poisoning

CO poisoning may occur if a car's engine is kept running inside a closed garage, an oil burner malfunctions, or an indoor wood fire in a poorly ventilated room generates carbon monoxide. In contrast to other poisonous fumes, carbon monoxide has no odor nor any noticeable color; unnoticed, it can kill quickly.

Suspect CO poisoning if you find the conditions mentioned above, and the victim has these symptoms: headache, weakness, dizziness, breathing difficulties, vomiting, and pink or red fingernails, skin, and lips.

WHAT YOU CAN DO

- Open all windows and doors; get the victim into fresh air.
- Call the police and fire department for rapid assistance, and investigation of the source of CO poisoning.
- Give artificial respiration and CPR if the person has no pulse, and is not breathing.
- Keep the victim covered and warm.

FOOD POISONING

Food contaminated by bacteria, poisonous mushrooms, or other ingested (eaten) poisonous substances may cause severe illness, and sometimes, death. Food poisoning is a common occurrence when foods are not cooked properly, or stored under adequate refrigeration. Bacteria such as Salmonella and other harmful organisms may multiply, causing severe and sometimes fatal cases of food poisoning if treatment is not promptly provided.

WHAT YOU CAN DO

- Take the victim to a hospital emergency room.
- Bring along a specimen of the poisoned food for analysis.

A PERSON HAS A NOSEBLEED—An emergency if bleeding is severe or does not stop—Call 911!

In young, otherwise healthy people, a nosebleed most often occurs as a result of an infection, inflammation or irritation of nasal tissues, injury, or a fracture (broken nose). Generally, the bleeding occurs only on one side of the nose.

WHAT YOU CAN DO

- Instruct the person to sit up.
- Apply pressure firmly to the bleeding nostril for five minutes to stop bleeding.
- Release pressure. If bleeding continues, apply pressure for another five minutes.
- Call 911 or take the person to a hospital emergency room if the above measures do not stop the bleeding.

A PERSON WITH INSECT BITES—No emergency unless victim is severely allergic—Then call 911!

- Apply ice to the area of the sting to reduce swelling, itching, or burning.
- Use an over-the-counter anti-itch medication; this usually clears up the bites within a few days.
- If there are signs of infection (persistent redness, swelling, or pus), obtain medical help.

A person stung by bees, wasps, or hornets

A healthy person not allergic to stings from these insects usually develops a painful red swelling after being stung, which disappears in a few days.

WHAT YOU CAN DO

- Scrape or tease (rather than pull) out the stinger, if present.
- Apply ice or cold compresses to lessen discomfort and reduce the swelling.
- Use an OTC antihistamine or hydrocortisone ointment to relieve pain, itching, and swelling.
- If swelling and discomfort persist, or infection develops at the site of the sting, seek medical help.

What you must do for a person who is allergic to bee, wasp, or hornet stings—Call 911!

- Immediately call for medical help. A person sensitive to such stings may die within minutes or even seconds from a hypersensitive reaction (anaphylactic shock), unless prompt measures are taken to reverse the reaction.
- Check a hypersensitive (highly allergic) person to see if he or she carries a kit containing a prefilled syringe with shock-preventive medication (epinephrine).
- Give, or have someone else give, the injection at once, then take the victim to the nearest hospital emergency room for further treatment.

A PERSON WITH TICK BITES—Not a major emergency, but may require medical examination

Ticks are tiny insects that infest deer, mice, and other animals such as dogs. These ticks may harbor an organism (*Borrelia Burgdorferi*), which is transmitted to humans by a tick bite. A bite from an infected tick may cause Lyme disease, with symptoms such as a red rash, arthritislike pains in the joints, and more serious symptoms involving the heart and nervous system.

WHAT YOU CAN DO

- After any outing such as a hike in the woods, search for and remove any tick with tweezers, and save it in a jar for identification.
- Check for development of a red rash at the site of the bite.
- If a rash or other symptoms (fever, headache, malaise) develop, take the victim for a medical checkup, diagnosis, and treatment.

A PERSON WITH A SEVERED FINGER, ARM, LEG, OR TOE—A major emergency—Call 911!

Accidents can result in the loss of a finger, toe, or limb.

WHAT YOU CAN DO
- Immediately look for and pick up, the severed part.
- Place the severed part in a clean plastic bag.
- Place this bag inside another plastic bag filled with ice.
- Immediately take the victim and the severed part to the nearest hospital emergency room. The shorter the time between the accident and the victim's arrival at the hospital, the greater the chance that the limb is viable (can be used again) and reattached to the body.
- As soon as emergency personnel arrive at the scene, immediately show them the severed part, to make sure appropriate action is taken at once.

A PERSON BITTEN BY AN ANIMAL (MAMMAL) OR HUMAN—Medical help always required. Not a life-threatening emergency unless there is heavy bleeding or a limb is severed—Then call 911!

WHAT YOU CAN DO
- For a minor scratch or bite: wash with soap and water, and cover with a clean cloth or sterile dressing.
- Get a medical examination, and treatment to prevent infection.
- For a severe or deep bite, call 911.
- Check for bleeding, presence of a pulse, and respirations.
- While waiting for medical help, take appropriate action for any injuries. *See* A person is bleeding heavily; A person is not breathing, Artificial respiration; Cardiac arrest, CPR.
- Keep victim warm.
- Hold the animal for possible examination for rabies.

A PERSON HAS A SNAKEBITE—Any snakebite is a major emergency—Call 911!

Many types of common snakes are not poisonous and do not bite. Poisonous snakes are found more frequently in tropical areas. Poisonous snakes of North America include the cottonmouth, coral, copperhead, and rattlesnakes. Learn about the types of snakes that live in your area, so you can recognize them in an emergency.

WHAT YOU CAN DO
- Keep the area of the bite below the level of the heart.

For a coral snakebite
- Keep the victim from moving, and wait for medical help.

For all other poisonous snakebites
- Apply a tightly wound bandage above the bite area, but don't cut off circulation.
- Prevent movement of the bitten area; keep the part as still as possible.
- Wash the bite area with soap and water. Do not use ice or cool compresses.
- Do not try to suck the snake venom out of the wound, regardless of the type of snakebite.

A CHILD OR ADULT WITH A FOREIGN BODY IN THE NOSE, EAR OR EYE— Not a major emergency, but may require medical follow-up

A child playing with a small toy may push it into an ear or nose. A foreign body in the eye may be dust, soot, other objects in the air, or an insect.

WHAT YOU CAN DO
Foreign body in the nose or ear
- Seek medical help if the object does not readily come out when the child blows his or her nose.
- Do not insert your finger or an instrument into the nose or ear to extricate a foreign body; you may cause injury and bleeding.
- If the object in the ear is a live insect, which produces acute discomfort: gently pour warm (never hot) oil in a slow stream from a small pitcher into the upturned ear, and check the return flow for the emerging insect. If it does not appear, and discomfort persists (the insect is still in the ear), seek medical help.

Foreign body in the eye
- Do not try to dislodge a foreign body or object from the eye, to avoid damage to delicate eye tissues, and possibly, to vision.
- Place a clean piece of cloth or sterile pad over the eye, and seek medical help.

A PERSON WITH CUTS OR SCRAPES—Not an emergency; seek medical help if bleeding persists or infection develops

Adults and children may sustain a cut (skin slit open, with minor bleeding) or a scrape (surface skin opened up due to contact with a sharp, rough, or uneven surface, resulting in no or minor bleeding). Bleeding is usually slight, and stops within one to three minutes.

WHAT YOU CAN DO
- If bleeding occurs, press a clean (sterile, if available) pad over the cut, and hold it for a few minutes.
- Once bleeding stops, apply a new sterile dressing to cover the wound and prevent inflammation or infection. Seek medical help if the wound does not look clean, pus appears, or bleeding does not stop.
- While waiting for medical help for a heavily bleeding wound, use First Aid for bleeding. *See* A person is bleeding heavily.

F

A PERSON EXPOSED TO CONTACT WITH POISONOUS PLANTS—Not a major emergency unless eyes or genitals are affected—Then call 911!

Many people are sensitive (allergic) to the irritating, oily substance that covers the leaves of certain plants, most commonly, Poison ivy, Poison oak, and Poison sumac.

Skin contact with these plants may later produce a severe itching or burning rash, which may develop into oozing blisters. Scratching these lesions is likely to spread the rash and blisters, causing intense itching and discomfort.

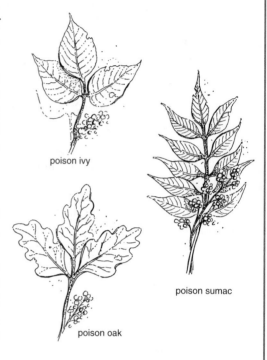

poison ivy

poison sumac

poison oak

WHAT YOU CAN DO

- Advise any person sensitive to these plants to become familiar with their appearance, and avoid contact.
- After skin contact immediately remove clothing, and wash affected areas at once with a strong soap (such as green soap) and water to remove the irritating substance, and possibly, prevent development of a rash.
- If a rash develops, spreads, becomes infected, or appears on the face or in the genital area, seek medical help for prompt treatment and relief of symptoms.

A PERSON WITH A BRUISE—Not a major emergency—Seek medical help if pain, swelling persist

A bruise occurs when a person falls, or sustains a blow, causing injury to the skin and tissues below. The bruise develops as a result of bleeding into tissues under the skin, causing a reddish-bluish-purplish tinge. The injury can cause significant pain, swelling, disability (a bruised ankle, for example), and take several weeks to heal.

WHAT YOU CAN DO

- Rest, and elevate the affected area.
- Apply cold, wet dressings or ice, 10 to 20 minutes every three or four hours for several days.
- Seek medical help if the swelling and pain persist, to check for a possible fracture.
- If a major bruise occurs on the face after a hard blow or fall, seek medical help. The victim's eyes, nose, and brain must be checked for injuries and treated promptly.

A PERSON WITH A FISHHOOK CAUGHT UNDER THE SKIN—Not a major emergency, but requires prompt medical follow-up

A fishhook caught under the skin is a painful, complicated yet common occurrence while fishing. It should be handled promptly, to cause a minimum of tissue damage, and to prevent infection.

WHAT YOU CAN DO

- Ask a doctor to remove the fishhook, and treat to avoid infection.
- If a doctor is not available, push the hook out through the skin, and cut off either the pointed end (hook end) or the straight end (shank end), as close to the skin as possible.
- Pull out the hook very carefully at the shorter end (hook or shank).
- Clean the wound, then apply a clean (or sterile) dressing.
- Obtain medical help. Do not neglect this: Treatment is necessary to prevent infection and other possible complications.

A PERSON WITH A PUNCTURE WOUND—Not a life-threatening emergency but requires medical treatment

A puncture wound may be superficial or deep. It may occur when a sharp, pointed object, such as a nail or an animal's tooth, penetrates the skin. Puncture wounds often occur in an unclean area, such as on the ground (earth or debris may get into the wound), or in an animal's mouth. Although the wound may be small, the chance of infection may be great. Prompt treatment to prevent infection is necessary.

WHAT YOU CAN DO

- Let the wound bleed. It does not usually bleed heavily, and the blood may wash out dirt, debris, and harmful bacteria.
- Cover the wound with a clean cloth or sterile dressing, and seek medical attention so that the victim can receive antibiotics and an injection of tetanus immune globulin, human (if he or she has not recently been immunized).

A PERSON WITH BLISTERS

Blisters (sacs of clear fluid or blood) may develop under the skin after an injury.

WHAT YOU CAN DO

The blister serves as a natural bandage; do not puncture or remove while intact. No treatment is usually needed.

A PERSON WITH A SPRAIN

Partial or complete tear of a ligament, the strong, fiberlike tissue that connects bones. A sprain may occur during a sports activity and may cause pain and swelling.

WHAT YOU CAN DO

Rest, an ice pack, elevation of the affected part, and a pain reliever such as aspirin or ibuprofen will reduce pain and start the healing process. An elastic bandage may help support the affected part. Depending on the severity of the sprain, healing may take from a few days to several weeks.

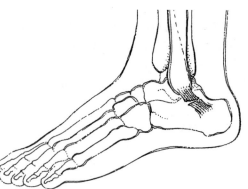

A PERSON WITH A STRAIN

Muscle discomfort or pain following excessive stretching or tearing of a muscle or its attached tendon. Strains occur in three degrees of severity:

First-degree strain: a slight tear with minimal loss of function.
Second-degree strain: a moderate tear with some loss of function.
Third-degree strain: a severe tear with nearly complete loss of function.

WHAT YOU CAN DO

A mild strain (first degree) is treated with Rest, Ice, Compression, and Elevation (RICE) until swelling and pain have decreased and function has returned. Second- and third-degree strains need to be checked and treated by a physician.

A PERSON HAS A SPLINTER—Not a major emergency unless the splinter is in an eye—In that case, call 911 or seek medical help promptly

A splinter is usually a sliver of wood, metal, or another substance sufficiently sharp to penetrate the skin and get stuck in or under it. A splinter is painful as well as potentially dangerous. If left in place, it may cause discomfort and infection.

WHAT YOU CAN DO

- If the splinter protrudes well out of the skin, pull it out with your (well-washed) hands, or with clean tweezers.
- If the splinter is located under, and near, the surface of the skin, heat (to sterilize) a razor blade and the tips of a pair of tweezers over a flame, then let them cool without touching any unclean surface.
- Make a tiny cut in the skin above the splinter with the razor blade, and use the tweezers to pull the splinter out.
- If the splinter is too large, or too deeply imbedded, cover the area with a clean cloth or sterile dressing, and seek medical help.